STOPPING SICKNESS

PREVENTION'S

FAMILY HEALTH LIBRARY™

STOPPING SICKNESS

How to Protect and Restore Your Good Health

by the Editors of
Prevention® Magazine

 Rodale Press, Emmaus, Pa.

Illustrations by Kathi Ember

Library of Congress Cataloging in Publication Data

Stopping sickness.

    (Prevention's family health library)
    1. Self-care, Health.   I. Prevention (Emmaus, Pa.)
II. Series. [DNLM: 1. Health. 2. Preventive Medicine—popular works.
WA 108 S883]
RA776.95.S76   1987   613   86-31322
ISBN 0-87857-707-6 paperback

2 4 6 8 10 9 7 5 3 1 paperback

NOTICE

Contents

CHAPTER 1

The Antiheadache Diet

An estimated 40 million Americans suffer from chronic headaches, some that defy aspirin and cold compresses, some so debilitating their victims lose jobs and families. Many desperate headache sufferers turn to high-powered painkillers or biofeedback techniques. But these days, an increasing number are learning to spell relief D-I-E-T.

It's a controversial remedy. There is little scientific evidence linking headaches to food. That puts doctors like Seymour Diamond, M.D., in a curious bind. Dr. Diamond, founder of the renowned Diamond Headache Clinic in Chicago and the National Migraine Foundation, has never been able to prove in the laboratory what he knows from his practice.

"As a researcher I have some doubts about the relationship of diet to headaches. As a clinician I have no doubts," he says. "Basically I'm a clinician who does research, so I have a very strong feeling that migraine sufferers are helped by diet—at least 25 to 30 percent of them are."

Migraine sufferers aren't the only people who can look to a dietary remedy. Some tension and muscular headaches, the dreaded "ice-cream headache," the headache of Chinese-restaurant syndrome may also respond to slight changes in eating habits.

Needless to say, there is no diet that cures them all. Each remedy is as individual as the headache, so "The Antiheadache Diet" isn't a diet at all but a set of guidelines, based on the advice of experts, that will help you determine a diet remedy that works for you.

1

The Migraine Headache

If you are susceptible to migraine headaches—severe vascular headaches that can leave you nauseous—certain foods can trigger pain. Wine (red in particular), aged cheese and chocolate all contain substances called amines, which can cause blood vessels to swell, triggering a headache. Nuts, salt and fresh baked bread are also known to bring on migraines in people with sensitive vascular systems.

Does this mean that migraine sufferers have to live on a boring diet of bland foods? Not necessarily. But they may have to alter their eating habits. Most headache experts have their own lists of "foods to avoid," but they agree that the best rule of thumb is: If it gives you a headache, don't eat it. It's not scientific, admits Joan Miller, Ph.D., a headache expert from Atlanta. "But my feeling is that the scientific evidence isn't as important as, 'Does it work?'"

Even if you consult a professional, it still is largely up to you to unravel your own personal headache mystery. But it might help to know a list of the most common suspects. Along with the ones we've mentioned, these include soy sauce, meats cured with nitrites, caffeinated beverages, foods containing the flavor enhancer monosodium glutamate, dairy products, broad beans such as limas and navy beans, citrus fruits, tomatoes, onions, pork, herring and other seafood, fresh wheat and yeast products, licorice and vinegar, except the white variety.

Most headache experts advise eliminating the amine-containing foods and experimenting with the others, eating one food at a time to determine if it figures in your headache. Of course, the method isn't foolproof. Some headaches don't appear until up to a day or two after the offending food is eaten. Some headaches aren't triggered by one but a combination of foods, or by food in tandem with stress.

"Many times you can get away with eating a certain food until you're under some stress, then the food plus the stress equals a migraine," says Dr. Miller. "I've had clients who've triggered a headache with a handful of peanuts eaten during a stressful time. Yet two weeks before they ate nuts and didn't get a headache."

Salt, like stress, is a subtle headache trigger. So says John Brainard, M.D., a surgeon from St. Paul, Minnesota, whose own migraines spurred him to write *Control of Migraines* (W. W. Norton & Company), the story of his dietary self-remedy.

Dr. Brainard noticed that when he ate salty foods, he was particularly susceptible to migraines. "Salt affects the blood vessels in such a way that it can make you very susceptible to other substances," he says.

In a study with migraine sufferers, Dr. Brainard gave patients small doses of salt. Fourteen of the 15 patients studied developed migraines. "When the salt hits the stomach lining, it stimulates the vagus nerve, which carries the impulse to the head, causing a headache."

A diet is not as restrictive as you may think. In fact, as diets go this one is truly painless. A typical day on the Diamond Headache Clinic diet starts with half a grapefruit, cereal or an egg, bran muffin with butter and jelly, and milk. Lunch might be roast turkey and the trimmings or cottage cheese and fruit. Dinner is a grilled hamburger on a bun, corn-on-the-cob and fresh melon.

The truth is, the migraine diet isn't all "foods to avoid." The "foods you can eat" list, provided here (see box), is far longer. But the key thing

---

Foods for the Headache Prone

This is the proverbial good news, foods that seem relatively safe for most headache sufferers. The selection was culled from the food lists provided by Seymour Diamond, M.D., of the Diamond Headache Clinic, Gunar Heuser, M.D., Ph.D., of the Beverly Hills Headache and Pain Medical Group, and John Brainard, M.D., author of *Control of Migraines*.

Dairy Products
Cottage cheese, cream cheese, yogurt (½ cup). Other cheeses may be tolerated if they are cooked in a dish like lasagna.

Desserts
Cakes, cookies, fruit pies, gelatin, tapioca. Avoid fresh yeast-raised products or those containing chocolate, nuts or raisins.

Fruits
Apples, apricots, bananas (½ a day), blueberries, cherries, citrus fruits (½ cup a day), cranberries, grapes peaches, pears.

Meats
Beef, chicken, duck, lamb, turkey, veal.

Vegetables
Artichokes, asparagus, beets, broccoli, carrots, cauliflower, celery, cucumbers, eggplant, green beans, leafy greens, mushrooms, parsnips, peas, potatoes, sprouts.

Miscellaneous
Commercial bread, carob, eggs, homemade salad dressings or commercial dressings in small amounts, homemade soups, salt-free snacks.

to note, says Dr. Diamond, is that foods—as far as possible—be minimally processed. That means soups, gravies and even salad dressings should be homemade. If you are a migraine sufferer, says Dr. Diamond, learn to read labels. No-no's like monosodium glutamate and excessive amounts of nitrites lurk in many canned or prepared foods.

The Food-Sensitivity Headache

She was 34 and for the last 10 years of her life she had a daily tension headache. At least, that's what her doctor called it. The other evidence was all there: temper outbursts, irritability, nervous tension, moodiness. The headache would go on for hours if she didn't take aspirin. Desperate, she sought help at the Institute of Health Psychology at North Texas State University in Denton.

There, psychologist Dan O'Banion, Ph.D., didn't discount the original diagnosis, but wasn't so sure her tension was psychological in origin. He placed her on an elimination diet, one that permitted her to eat only one food at a time. For the first time in a decade, the patient had several successive headache-free days—days, not coincidentally, when she didn't eat corn, wheat, milk products, cola drinks and tea.

"Hers was a tension headache," says Dr. O'Banion, "but the tension was caused by her food sensitivity. Much of the increased stress load on people like this is due to diet. Their bodies become toxic and it makes them susceptible to even small psychological problems."

Though relatively simple to pinpoint, food-sensitivity headaches aren't always simple to cure. Often the victims are sensitive to their favorite foods. The fact is, the psychologist says, many food-sensitive people become addicted to the food they're sensitive to. They get a "high" when they eat it, and crash when they don't. The headache they experience when they don't get their "food fix" is a symptom of withdrawal, Dr. O'Banion says. Some people even wake up several times a night, unable to sleep until they eat their particular addictive food.

The only diet remedy for this particular headache is similar to that for a migraine: Eat only fresh foods and use an elimination test to determine which foods trigger your particular headache. The food-withdrawal headache usually occurs two to three hours after the offending food is eaten, says Dr. O'Banion. You might have to suffer with it for several days, he warns, until you shake the addictive cycle.

The Hypoglycemic Headache

When the sugar content of the blood drops, blood vessels swell, causing vascular headaches such as migraines, says Dr. Diamond in a book he co-authored with Judi Diamond-Falk, *Advice from the Diamond Headache Clinic* (International Universities Press). These headaches can be avoided if you eat several small meals a day, have a protein snack before bed so your blood sugar doesn't dwindle by morning, and avoid simple-carbohydrate, high-sugar foods that cause a rapid rise and fall in blood-sugar levels.

The Hunger Headache

Similar to the hypoglycemic headache, this one is also caused by a drop in blood sugar, says Dr. Diamond. The remedy is simple: Eat at least three well-balanced meals a day.

The Hangover Headache

This headache is avoidable. Simply don't drink to excess. But if you expect to overindulge, says Dr. Diamond, there is a way to lessen the pain. Eating fruit or honey, even drinking tomato juice, can reduce the impact of a hangover headache. Fructose helps the body metabolize ethyl alcohol, he says.

The Caffeine and Caffeine-Withdrawal Headaches

This is a case of damned if you do and damned if you don't. Caffeine can cause a headache if you drink it and if you suddenly stop drinking it.

A strong stimulant, caffeine can make you so edgy you develop a tension headache. It can keep you awake, inviting the dull throb of fatigue. It can also raise your blood pressure, which can give you a dull, pounding headache or increase the frequency of your migraines.

Caffeine is also a vasoconstrictor—it makes your blood vessels contract. They can adapt quite readily to this semiconstricted state if you're a habitual caffeine drinker. But if you decide to go cold turkey, vessels swell, leaving you with a dull withdrawal headache that can be cured only by more caffeine—or time and a painkiller. The best remedy, says Dr. Diamond, is to gradually wean yourself from caffeine.

The Poor-Nutrition Headache

Many headache sufferers simply don't take good care of themselves, says Dr. Miller. Many bear an uncanny resemblance to the typical type-A personality: busy fussbudgets who'll forgo meals and family affairs to work, work, work. The missed meals often mean a loss of the B complex vitamins, which can leave these individuals edgy and prone to headaches.

The best cure for this headache is prevention, Dr. Miller says. A well-balanced diet and evenly spaced meals—that means no snacks on the run—will keep your body healthy and the headaches away.

The Hot-Dog Headache

The culprit isn't that familiar *cuisine de ballpark* per se, it's the nitrites used in the curing process that give the meat that appetizing red color. Nitrites are found in everything from lunch meat to bacon and there is a cure for this cure. Just add cured meats to your "foods to avoid" list.

Chinese-Restaurant Syndrome

Some people don't get hungry an hour after eating Chinese food. They get a headache. Monosodium glutamate, or MSG, can trigger this reaction, which also includes a feeling of tightness in the chest and a burning sensation in the face, neck and torso. You don't have to give up Chinese food. Many restaurants don't add this flavor enhancer and most would be happy to leave it out of your dish if you ask.

According to Rosemary Dudley, executive vice president of the Migraine Foundation of Canada, MSG headaches are most pronounced if you eat on an empty stomach, so before your Chinese dinner, eat a roll or a salad. Also, try to avoid starting your meal with soup, which can contain more MSG than the vegetable and meat entrées.

Be forewarned: MSG is also in some processed and prepared foods. If you don't already read food labels, start. You might save yourself a headache later on.

The Ice-Cream Headache

You've just taken a big bite of butter almond and an intense, dull pain radiates throughout your head. Not what you had in mind, was it? Exactly what causes an ice-cream headache isn't known. But, according to Dr. Diamond, the pain may be a response of the warm tissues of the mouth to the cold substance. Two nerves there carry impulses—including pain—to the head, which explains why the headache is generalized in the head and throat.

If you're a victim, there's a way to eat ice cream that won't bring on a headache. Simply allow small amounts of ice cream, or other cold substances, to melt or warm up in the mouth so that the mouth cools slowly, advises Dr. Diamond.

CHAPTER 2

Super Sleep from A to Z-Z-Z

J ane knows exactly when her sleep troubles started. She was a young mother with children aged one, three and five. When they all became sick at the same time, she would lie awake at night listening for their cries or coughs, fearful of missing a cue that could affect the outcome of their illnesses.

In a few weeks' time, all the children had completely recovered, but Jane's pattern of nighttime wakefulness had been set. And it persisted for years, along with worrying about her children's health and her lack of sleep.

"Insomnia, whether it's trouble falling asleep or trouble staying asleep, can often be traced back to a single disturbing event," says Michael Stevenson, Ph.D., director of the insomnia clinic at Holy Cross Hospital in Mission Hills, California. "The event may pass as in Jane's case, but if the worry continues it can lead to sleep anxiety and more insomnia."

You worry because you can't sleep and then you can't sleep because you're worried. Sound familiar? It should, since half the population experiences at least occasional sleep difficulties at any given time. But whether your insomnia is chronic or occasional, has lasted for one week or 20 years, there are no hopeless cases, according to the sleep experts we consulted. If you are having trouble sleeping, maybe you haven't considered all the factors that can affect the quantity and quality of your sleep. Our list of sleep tips is intended to open your eyes now so that you can close them more easily later.

Design Your Bedroom for Maximum Sleep Comfort

• Room temperature between 64° and 66°F is most conducive to sound sleep, says Elliot Richard Phillips, M.D., medical director of the Sleep Disorders Center at Holy Cross Hospital and a colleague of Dr. Stevenson. Too cold and you'll be fumbling for covers. Too hot and you have restless, light sleep.

• Keep your bedroom as quiet as possible. If you live near an airport or superhighway, don't despair. You can mask offending sounds with a device that generates "white noise" (soothing background sounds such as a simulated rain, surf or waterfalls), says Jerrold S. Maxmen, M.D., author of *A Good Night's Sleep* (W. W. Norton and Company).

• Try sleeping on air or water—an air mattress or water bed. And replace any mattress that's saggy or lumpy.

• A fleecy woolen mattress pad placed between the mattress and bottom sheet can have a positive effect on sleep, according to an Australian study. The volunteers who slept on the woolen pad reported less tossing and turning and felt better in the morning than those who slept on a conventional pad (*Medical Journal of Australia,* January 21, 1984).

• Wool blankets are better able to regulate skin and body temperature than acrylic blankets, resulting in a more comfortable sleeping environment.

• Get rid of overly soft, fluffy pillows. They can cause neck stiffness, which disrupts sleep.

Associate Your Bedroom with Relaxation and Sleep

• Don't use your bedroom as an office, says Thomas J. Coates, Ph.D., co-director of the behaviorial medicine unit at the University of California School of Medicine in San Francisco. "One woman I counseled had done just that. She had re-entered the job market and had placed her desk in her bedroom. Every time she saw it there she would get uptight and depressed. When she placed her desk in another room—away from her bedroom—her insomnia disappeared."

"I used to have my personal computer and exercise equipment in my bedroom," says Dr. Phillips. "I spent many wakeful hours in the bedroom doing things that were not restful, not conducive to sleep."

• Don't use the bedroom as a battlefield. Another patient of Dr. Coates's said that the bedroom was the only room where she and her husband could argue without the children hearing. "Now they use the garage and she is sleeping again," says Dr. Coates.

• Practice relaxation techniques or self-hypnosis in the bedroom. (There are many good self-help books to assist you.)

• If you haven't fallen asleep after 20 to 30 minutes, get up and leave the bedroom. This way you won't associate your bedroom with sleeplessness.

• Leave worries outside the bedroom by giving yourself a specific worry time, advises Dr. Stevenson. That's when you mull over the day's activities and play your next moves.

If your brain still feels cluttered with details, write them all down on a piece of paper. That way your head doesn't have to remember them.

• Love your place of sleep. Decorate your bedroom in your favorite colors and fabrics. Bring in objects (like photographs and souvenirs) that help you recall the most pleasant times in your life.

How Diet Can Affect Sleep

• L-tryptophan, an amino acid naturally found in protein foods (milk products, tuna, turkey and peanuts are especially good sources) has already been proved effective for people with *mild* insomnia. Now a new study from Switzerland has shown that chronic insomniacs can benefit from this nutrient as well. The 40 patients who participated in the experiment took L-tryptophan on a three-day-on, four-day-off schedule (two grams per day) for about four months. By the end of the study, half the patients said they were sleeping normally, while another 30 percent reported that their sleep patterns were "much improved." Even at a two-year followup, most of the patients were still sleeping well even though they were no longer taking the L-tryptophan.

• Eating carbohydrates along with the L-tryptophan may increase the effectiveness of the nutrient, according to Richard Wurtman, Ph.D., of the Center for Brain Sciences and Metabolism at the Massachusetts Institute of Technology. After a high-carbohydrate meal is eaten, insulin is released. This hormone helps clear the way for tryptophan to be carried to the brain. Once there, it is converted to serotonin, a neurotransmitter that is involved in producing sleeplessness.

• Avoid foods containing simple sugars (such as candy bars or cookies) at bedtime, advises Dr. Stevenson. "They often make people feel 'hyped-up!' Instead have milk and a banana or even a small tuna sandwich, which contains both complex carbohydrates and L-tryptophan."

• Don't go to bed hungry, even if you are dieting. Hunger pangs and the feeling of emptiness in the stomach can lead to restlessness and a poor night's sleep.

• Don't go to bed right after a mammoth meal, either. It's hard to sleep when your digestive system is working overtime.

How Drugs Affect Sleep

• Give up cigarettes along with caffeine. Studies have shown that the nicotine found in cigarettes can adversely affect your sleep. In one study, researchers found that nonsmokers fell asleep after about 30 minutes, while it took smokers an average of 44 minutes. In a separate experiment, heavy smokers, who agreed to quit all at once, decreased the total time spent awake by 45 percent, in the first three nights alone (*Science,* February, 1980).

• Prescription sleeping pills are not recommended by any of the experts we spoke to. "Sleeping pills such as Valium or Dalmane produce poor sleep quality while you take them," explains Dr. Phillips.

"But you get into even more trouble when you try to quit. There's a physiological withdrawal your system must go through which causes insomnia. You can see how people get hooked."

• Over-the-counter (OTC) sleeping medications are equally frowned upon. "There's a withdrawal problem from these preparations as well", says Dr. Phillips. "What's more, the main ingredient in the OTC's is actually an antihistamine, which may produce some potentially serious side effects if used for prolonged periods. It can cause glaucoma to worsen, produce irregular heartbeats and urinary problems. These medications should not be used casually."

• Diuretics (drugs which remove excess fluid from your tissues) may disturb sleep because they cause frequent trips to the bathroom.

• Antibiotics, or any prescription medication for that matter, have the potential to disturb sleep. If your sleep problems seem to coincide with taking a new medication, consult your doctor or pharmacist about this side effect.

Your Situation Levels Affect Sleep

• Situational insomnia is the name given to short periods of sleeplessness which occur before, during or after times of great stress. Any number of events—both good and bad—can trigger it. Buying a house, losing a job, an impending trip are typical causes. The good news is that this state of hyperarousal rarely lasts longer than three weeks. The only treatment needed, says Dr. Phillips, is reassurance that when you calm down your sleep will return to normal.

• Boredom, perhaps the opposite of situational insomnia, can also cause loss of sleep, according to Dr. Coates. His study found that poor sleepers spent more time shopping, relaxing and watching TV, and thought more about going to bed. The good sleepers were more mentally and physically active. They spent more time working, talking and doing chores.

• Increase social contacts. Isolated people are poor sleepers, says Dr. Coates. Those with a social support system sleep better and are also less depressed, which in itself helps relieve insomnia.

• Become other-preoccupied instead of self-preoccupied. Get involved in a project or do volunteer work to get your thoughts off yourself. "Often," says Dr. Stevenson, "insomnia can be traced back to within one week of retirement. Isolation, boredom, loss of social contacts and preoccupation with self all hit at once. Sleep goes right out the window. Sometimes we have to get the person to go back to work."

Refine Your Sleep Routine

• Don't go to bed until you are sleepy. Do something relaxing until you feel tired.

• Get up the same time each morning, every day of the week, regardless of when you went to bed, when you fell asleep or how many hours of sleep you've gotten. "This is one of the most important rules of all," points out Dr. Phillips. "By getting up at the same time every morning, no matter how poor the night's sleep has been, you accomplish two things. The body's daily or circadian rhythm is reset, so that it expects to get up from sleep at the same time tomorrow, and all other sleep and wake cycles are synchronized."

• If you get up earlier you force yourself to get sleepy earlier. Suppose your natural sleepiness doesn't occur until one in the morning — too late for a nine-to-fiver. By forcing yourself to wake up an hour earlier every morning, you can reset your body clock and shift your sleep/wake schedule to one more conducive to your workaday lifestyle.

• Oversleeping on the weekends is a sure way to mess up a body clock, says Dr. Maxmen. You not only become less alert after too much sleep, but you reduce the number of wakeful hours, making it more difficult to fall asleep the next night.

• Don't take a daytime nap no matter how groggy you may feel. For most people, a daytime snooze will decrease the quality and quantity

5 Sleep Myths That Can Keep You Awake

1. Everybody needs eight hours of uninterrupted sleep to feel their best. Not so, says Dr. Phillips. "Some people do well on four. Others need ten. Recognize and accept individual sleeping patterns. Remember, too, that as you get older you require even less sleep."

2. A glass of wine or a hot toddy at bedtime will help you sleep. "Initially it does induce sleepiness," Dr. Stevenson told us. "But about two to three hours after drinking you go through alcohol withdrawal, which actually arouses the nervous system to a higher level than before. Too much wine with dinner and you may be unable to fall asleep at bedtime. If the wine is drunk at bedtime, you may fall asleep easily, only to find yourself wide awake in the middle of the night."

"I can't tell you how many patients we see whose sleep problems completely disappear after they stop having wine with dinner," adds Dr. Phillips.

3. You should go to bed extra early so you can be well rested before an important day. This just doesn't work and, in fact, will most likely have the opposite effect. You'll find yourself tossing and turning and getting even more aroused if you try to go to sleep before your body's regular turn-in time.

4. Vigorous exercise right before bedtime will really knock you out. On the contrary, says Dr. Phillips, strenuous exercise at bedtime will overstimulate the cardiovascular and nervous systems and make it difficult for you to unwind and relax.

However, consistent or daily exercise done in the late afternoon or early evening will indeed extend and deepen sleep, says Dr. Maxmen. But exercise moderation, too, or you'll find yourself kept awake with the aches and pains of overexertion.

5. Sex before bedtime is the best natural sleep inducer. "It is for some folks," says Dr. Coates. "But for many others it's a real energizer. If you're in the latter group, it may be necessary for you to rearrange your love-making times to the morning or early evening."

of sleep at night. Get some fresh air or take a walk until you get your second wind.

• Develop your own sleep ritual if you don't already have one. Do you close all the windows, check that the doors are locked, wash up, read before bed? Sleep rituals prepare you for bed psychologically as well as physically and should be continued even when you're away from home.

• Sleeping alone after years of having a partner can cause sleep disturbances. Dr. Coates has had some success in treating elderly widowed patients by advising them to get a cat or dog to cuddle.

• When taking a business trip (notorious for disturbing sleep patterns) take along your favorite pillow and the pajamas you wear at home. Have the operator give you a wake-up call to eliminate the fear of oversleeping.

• Emphasize good sleep habits in your children. "I've seen quite a few people whose sleep problems began in childhood," Dr. Stevenson told us. "Their parents didn't regulate their bed and wake-up times and consequently they are having problems as adults. Sleep is a learned act (many aspects of sleep are learned). It's important for a baby to have a definite sleep/wake schedule. Of course, there should be some flexibility, but it's a disservice to children to let them stay up till all hours and sleep till all hours. The real world operates on a regular schedule."

CHAPTER 3

Virus Busters

The average American, says the U.S. Public Health Service, experiences more than 200 viral infections during his or her lifetime. There are vaccines against a few of the scarier viruses—polio, for example, and measles—but there has never been a universal vaccine against colds and flu. So let's take stock of the natural virus busters that we have at our disposal.

One of them is zinc. It's long been recognized that zinc in the diet is necessary for a strong immune response. Without zinc, the body's germ-fighting white blood cells would malfunction and wounds wouldn't heal. But a group of researchers in Austin, Texas, have reported that zinc lozenges dissolved in the mouth can have a remarkably direct effect on the duration of colds. Medical researchers at the Clayton Foundation Biochemical Institute in Austin set up an experiment to see whether zinc lozenges could cure colds. Sixty-five people with colds took part in the experiment. Thirty-seven were given zinc gluconate tablets every other waking hour, and the rest received a placebo. Every subject carefully recorded his or her headaches, sneezes and coughs for a week.

The results were almost too good to be true. "In the zinc-treated group, sizable numbers of subjects became asymptomatic within hours," the researchers said. Within a day, one-fifth of the zinc group was fully recuperated. None of the placebo group recovered that fast. The average length of a cold was 3.9 days in the zinc group, compared to 10.8 days in the placebo group (*Antimicrobial Agents and Chemotherapy*, January, 1984).

14

But the zinc worked only when it was dissolved like a hard candy instead of being swallowed like a pill. That's because the zinc ions possibly came into direct contact with the viruses in the respiratory tract.

"We hope this will be a big step toward controlling the common cold," says Donald R. Davis, Ph.D., of the Clayton Foundation, who analyzed the experiment. "The next step is to find out exactly how much zinc should be used and how often it needs to be applied. You have to remember that we're talking about treating an existing cold, not preventing one," he added, "although it's possible that if your diet is rich in zinc, you would suffer fewer colds." Dr. Davis adds that several people dropped out of his experiment because they didn't like the taste of the lozenges. And not all zinc supplements are equally effective. In fact, Dr. Davis notes that the zinc treatment needs much further study before it can be recommended to the public.

Vitamin C and interferon are two more virus busters. There has been so much talk about synthesizing interferon and marketing it as a drug that we tend to forget that it is also a natural substance, which protects us against invaders 24 hours a day without costing us a cent. Whenever a healthy cell comes under attack by a virus, the cell manufacturers interferon and sends it off in all directions, like an army of Paul Reveres, warning neighboring cells to defend themselves. Once a nearby cell is merely touched by interferon, it becomes incapable of doing what the virus most wants it to do—namely, to convert its nucleus into a virus factory. A cell that's immunized by interferon may still be invaded by a virus, but no new viruses will be born. To borrow computer terminology, the virus will be unable to replace the cell's genetic software with its own.

All cells have the ability to produce interferon, but we can give that ability a boost by increasing our intake of vitamin C. Benjamin Siegel, Ph.D., a professor of pathology at the Oregon Health Sciences University, has found that mice given vitamin C supplements have higher levels of interferon in their blood than mice who receive no extra vitamin C. "It's possible that vitamin C stimulates the increased production of interferon by the affected cell," he says.

The body has another built-in virus buster: fever. Both flu viruses and cold viruses like it relatively cool. They flourish where the temperature is between 86° and 95°F. The body core is too hot for them, but the nasal passages cooled by inhalation, are just right. Heat up the nostrils with fever, however, and the viruses shrivel up and die.

Here's how fever works. When viruses or bacteria invade the body, the germ-fighting white blood cells release a protein called pryogen, which in Greek means "heat-producing." Pryogen tells the brain to raise the body's temperature from 98.6° to about 102°F. Experiments with animals have shown that when the temperature in the body goes up, the amount of live viruses in the nasal passages goes down.

Fever is difficult to control, however, so other methods for heating up the nose and throat have been suggested. A steam bath followed by a hot toddy is one traditional cure. Inhaling warm water vapor is another. One researcher has suggested that regular exercise promotes the release of pryogen, which keeps the body temperature high for several hours after the workout is over (*Physician and Sportsmedicine*, March, 1983).

Mind Power vs. Virus Power

People who have friends they can turn to in times of stress have more resistance to viral infections than people who are lonely.

In England, a few years ago, a group of psychologists wanted to find what effect, if any, the emotional events in a person's life might have on the severity of their colds. Would a man's head cold, for instance, be worse if his love affair had just ended? Would a woman's cold be milder if she'd just gotten a new job? The psychologists had a hunch that emotional lows go hand in hand with bad colds. But they weren't sure.

To find out, they recruited 52 men and women between the ages of 18 and 49—housewives, students, working people and professionals. Each one went through a battery of psychological tests and personality inventories. How introverted or extroverted were they? Had they been seeing a lot of people lately or had they gone off by themselves? How were they spending their leisure time?

They came the ultimate sacrifice. Each volunteer agreed to "catch a cold." They were all inoculated with common cold viruses and then confined to a hospital ward for ten days of close observation. The amount of virus present in their mucus was precisely noted, as were their sneezes, coughs and even the number of tissues they used to blow their noses.

At its conclusion, the experiment yielded "clear evidence of a psychosomatic component in colds." People who were outgoing and extroverted had milder colds than people who were introverted. And it appeared that people who had recently withdrawn from their friends and hobbies had the worst cold symptoms of all. But the clearest finding was that people who had gone through the most drastic life changes—either for the better or worse, it didn't seem to matter—had the highest virus levels in their respiratory tracts and therefore the worst infections (*Journal of Psychosomatic Research,* vol. 24, 1980).

Relax Away That Virus Attack

Loneliness and stress sometimes combine to put a double whammy on our resistance to viral infection. At Ohio State University a group of researchers decided that they'd heard too many "anecdotes" about the way stress brings on herpes virus attacks, which produce cold sores and fever blisters. They wanted proof.

The researchers took three blood samples from a group of 49 medical students to determine the level of herpes virus antibodies in their blood. A high level of antibodies, in this case, would indicate a diminished resistance to the virus. Blood samples were taken a month before final exams, on the first day of final exams, and during the first week back from summer vacation. The students also took a psychological test to measure how lonely they were.

Resistance to the virus turned out to be highest after the vacation, when the students were relaxed. And the lonelier students had significantly less resistance to the virus than the more gregarious students had.

In a very similar experiment, also at Ohio State, a group of 30 residents of a retirement home was divided into thirds. One group received relaxation training three times a week, the second group received individual "social contact" three times a week, and the last group had no contact with the researchers. Those who learned to relax, it turned out, experienced a 32 percent rise in their white blood cell levels. Those who received social contact enjoyed an 18 percent rise. The no-contact group suffered a 6 percent loss of white blood cells, and its members showed the least resistance to herpes virus infections (*Proceedings of the Society of Behaviorial Medicine,* May 23-26, 1984).

People who have type-A personalities—who are compulsively achievement oriented and live in a chronic state of self-imposed stress—also seem to come down with more respiratory-tract infections than do type-B personalities, who don't push themselves as much.

At Colorado State University, 30 type-A male and female students and a similar group of type-B students were asked to recall how many viral colds they'd had in the preceding year. By a significant margin, the type A's reported more colds than the type B's. That came as a surprise, because, if anything, type A's can be expected to underreport any behavior that might make them appear weak. They also tend to ignore their symptoms instead of staying in bed and taking aspirin and vitamin C. To explain why type A's get more colds, the researchers suggested that the same body chemicals that type A's use to rev themselves up—called catecholamines—also have, as a side effect, the ability to reduce the body's resistance to infection (*Journal of Human Stress,* June, 1982).

John Mills, M.D., a professor of medicine and microbiology at the University of California School of Medicine in San Francisco, offers a few more tips on how to avoid cold and flu viruses:

• Colds are most often "caught" when someone rubs his or her nose or eye after having touched the hand of an infected person who has just touched his nose. Keeping hands away from noses is a good idea.

• Coughing and sneezing are definite signs of a cold, but they are much less likely to pass a cold from one person to another. Sneezes and coughs contain very little virus.

• Taking aspirin reduces the symptoms of a cold, but increases the amount of virus in the nose. If you take aspirin, be extra careful not to touch your nose.

• Merely rinsing your hands under water for 30 seconds effectively washes away any viruses that might be on them.

• Don't worry about venturing out into the wintry weather. There's no evidence that cold weather alone will give you a virus infection or even worsen the one you may already have.

CHAPTER 4

Instant Help for
Everyday Aches and Pains

Home-remedy painkillers? They work like any other painkiller—giving you instant comfort rather than permanent cure. In the long run, you'll probably have to undertake an exercise program to make your aching back fit again and deal with the stress that brought on your headache in the first place. But you can do that once today's pain is gone.

What's the magic? No magic. Just some good commonsense advice from doctors and therapists who deal with pain every day. You'll have to learn when heat helps and when ice is your treatment of choice. You may have to make some lifestyle changes, learn about massage and acupressure and add a few pain-relieving products to your shopping list. But you can administer this brand of first aid without fear—and for just about any common ache or pain from head to toe.

A cautionary note: If pain is your enemy, consider it a friendly one. It's your body's way of telling you something is wrong. You don't want to mask the causes of pain. If you have a serious condition or if pain persists, see a physician. Only minor aches and pains should be treated at home.

Headache

• If your face feels tight, your nose is full and your headache seems to be enveloping your face as well, you probably have a sinus headache. Steam or moist heat may help. If you can't get to a steam bath, make your own. Sit in the bathroom with the shower running hot and hard. Or

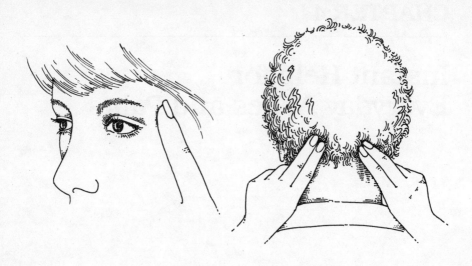

try a warm pack across the eyes and cheekbones. Take a fluffy, thick washcloth and soak it in warm water. After you wring it out, apply it to the area that hurts. When it cools off, warm it up and reapply for about ten minutes. A steam vaporizer can be of inestimable value when a sinus headache hits.

• According to migraine expert Seymour Diamond, M.D., you can run away from a headache. Running, at least in theory, increases the production of endorphins, the body's natural painkillers. Dr. Diamond, executive director of the National Migraine Foundation and director of the Diamond Headache Clinic in Chicago, thinks these natural painkillers may be responsible for the relief migraine sufferers experience after jogging. For people who find running relaxing, he says, it could also relieve a muscle tension headache.

• When headache strikes, use your thumbs. Howard D. Kurland, M.D., author of *Quick Headache Relief without Drugs* (William Morrow and Company), advises headache sufferers to use acupressure, a version of acupuncture without the needles. The pressure of a blunt thumbnail on certain nerve points seems to relieve pain, says Dr. Kurland. Common headaches respond to pressure on two main points on the head and two accessory points on the hands.

The first main point is by the eye. Find a point halfway between the outer corner of the eye and outer end of the eyebrow. (See illustration above, left.) Your finger will be on a ridge of bone, which is the outer edge of your eye socket. Move one finger's breadth back toward

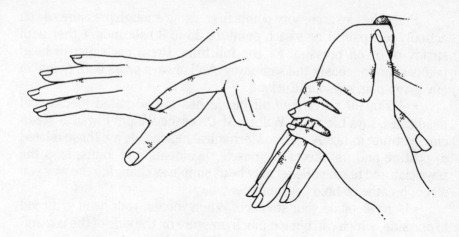

the ear and you'll be touching a small depression, which is the first main point.

The second main point is at the base of the skull. Find the bony ridge behind the ear known as the mastoid bone. Then find a large muscular groove at midpoint in the back of your neck. Halfway between the two, on each side of the neck, there will be a smaller groove between two muscles. Run your thumbnail up the small groove until you come to the base of the skull. Push inward and upward with some force into the groove and against the bone. (See illustration on page 20, right.) That's main point two.

Find the first accessory point by spreading out your hand so the web of the thumb is stretched out. The point is in that triangle of skin between your thumb and index finger on the back of your hand. It's near the bone that runs from the knuckle of your index finger back to the wrist, on the thumb side of the bone and closer to the index finger than to the thumb. (See illustration above, left.) You should know you've found it when you press hard. Usually, pressure on these points hurts, just as if you'd struck your funny bone.

The second accessory point is on the wrist. Spread your thumb out and as far back as it will go. Two long tendons will stand out. Where they vanish into the wrist there will be a hollow space. Immediately above this hollow space is a small bone protuberance. Two fingers' width above this is a small depression, which is accessory point two. (See illustration above, right.)

Press the two accessory points first, using enough pressure so you actually feel pain. Press each point for 25 to 30 seconds, either with steady or on-off pressure for the full time. Press each pair of head points simultaneously the same way. And always press both points in any given pair, says Dr. Kurland.

• About 90 percent of all headaches are so-called mechanical headaches, says Lionel A. Walpin, M.D., of the Walpin Physical Medicine Institute in Los Angeles. Mechanical headaches are those related to posture and its effects on muscle, ligaments and joints, says the physician and teacher. Relief may be as simple as changing the way you sleep, breathe or hold your tongue.

• Don't sleep on your stomach. When you do, your head is turned to one side, which can put too much pressure on the side of the jaw and upper neck, causing a headache. Dr. Walpin has even co-developed a pillow—called the Wal·Pil·O—a four-in-one cervical pillow that, among other things, discourages you from sleeping in that awkward stomach position and allows your muscles to relax, leading to more restful sleep.

• Breathe through your nose, not your mouth. Not only will you draw more air into your lungs, you'll hold your head and shoulders in a better posture in relation to your body. "You shouldn't use your neck and upper chest to breathe," says Dr. Walpin. "They're not designed for that. If you do, they'll become sore and refer pain to your head and shoulders."

Facial Pain and Toothaches

• Look for a mechanical cause. Do you wear sunglasses? A researcher at the University of Arizona College of Medicine found that three young women who had complained of numbness, burning and pain beneath their eyes had only one thing in common: They had all begun wearing sunglasses recently. He theorized that the sunglasses caused the problem because they're large and can irritate the facial nerve.

• Consider trying tryptophan. Researchers at Temple University in Philadelphia found that three grams of tryptophan administered in conjunction with a high-carbohydrate, low-fat and low-protein diet relieved facial pain and increased pain tolerance among 30 chronic pain patients. Tryptophan is an amino acid that is a precursor of serotonin, a neurotransmitter in the brain that increases the effectiveness of the body's endorphins.

• At McGill University in Montreal scientists discovered they could relieve toothaches with an ice massage . . . but not by massaging anywhere near the teeth. They treated patients suffering from acute dental pain by massaging the web between the thumb and index finger of the hand on the same side as the dental pain (that's the very spot where you apply acupressure for a headache). Ice massage decreased the intensity of the dental pain by half in most of the patients (*Canadian Medical Association Journal,* January 26, 1980).

Neck Pain

• If your neck aches in the morning, the culprit may be your sleeping habits, says James Fries, M.D., author of *Arthritis: A Comprehensive Guide* (Addison-Wesley Publishing Company) and co-author of *Take Care of Yourself* (Addison-Wesley Publishing Company). Sleep on a firm mattress and throw away your pillow. For the pain, try heat: a nice hot shower, hot compresses or a heating pad. To give your neck support, take a bath towel, fold it lengthwise so that it's about four inches wide and wrap your neck with it, securing it with a safety pin or tape. This, says Dr. Fries, will clear up "nearly half of all neck pain problems" by simply supporting the neck and reminding you not to turn too quickly or too far.

Shoulder Pain

• Usually this common pain comes from the soft tissues near the joint and not from the bones or joints themselves, says Dr. Fries. Gentle heat usually helps (though sometimes so does a cold pack) followed by exercises to help maintain mobility in the joint.
• A good pain-relieving shoulder exercise is the pendulum swing: Lean over so that your arm hangs like a pendulum and swing it around in ever-increasing circles.
• To ease shoulder pain, it might also help to improve your posture. The shoulder is anatomically susceptible to fatigue. Try to relax, not tense your neck and upper back muscles when you're under stress.

Tennis Elbow

• Needless to say, you're probably going to have to improve your technique and follow a few other rules laid down by New York physical therapist Eileen Shepherd: Don't buy a prestrung racket (they're too tight); use a two-handed backhand; avoid frequent change from slow clay to faster asphalt (or vice versa); keep your elbow bent and keep your eye on the ball. For the immediate pain, physicians recommend heat and range-of-motion exercises as your best bet.

Side Stitches

• You're out for a short run when suddenly there's a painful catch just below your rib cage. It makes you stop and, probably instinctively, you do exactly what you're supposed to do: Breathe it away. You change your breathing pattern from deep rhythmic breathing to shallow quick breathing or vice versa. Breathing from your diaphragm should make you less susceptible to this minor ache.

Back Pain

• An estimated seven million people are treated for back pain on any given day. In fact, it's been calculated that 80 percent of us will have a bout with backache at some time in our lives. The causes of back pain are legion, as are the cures. You may have to try several, or a combination, before you find a remedy for yourself. What you don't want to do is rely on muscle relaxants and painkillers, says Dr. Fries. They may get you moving around, but you're also likely to reinjure your back when the pain is masked. Therefore, medication is best used when accompanied by the first rule of back care: rest.

• If it's an injury that's laying your back low, don't reach for the comfort of a heating pad, as most people do, says James J. Irrgang, R.P.T., director of the Center for Sports Medicine at the National Hospital for Orthopedics and Rehabilitation in Arlington, Virginia. For trauma, reach for ice. "It helps reduce inflammation and eliminate pain, and prevents much of the swelling from occurring," says the physical therapist. "Heat can make all those things—inflammation, pain and swelling—much worse, especially right after the injury." An ice "popsicle" applied to the sore area for 15 minutes every four to six hours can effectively anesthetize the muscle spasm that accompanies back injuries such as muscle strain. (To make your ice pop, freeze a paper cup filled with water and then tear off the upper half. Peel the remainder as the ice melts.)

• For the days following an injury or if your back problem is limited to pain and stiffness, especially on awakening, heat is your answer. A hot bath or shower, heating pad, hot-water bottle, even hot wet towels help.

• The worst enemy of your back may be your mattress. Many back sufferers find a nice firm mattress prevents the pain and stiffness that comes with morning. Others prefer a waterbed. A ¾-inch-thick piece of plywood under the mattress is a do-it-yourself mattress firmer.

• Change positions frequently, not only while you're sleeping but while you're working too. Remaining in one place too long can turn your sore muscles to stone.

• Correct your posture. Many backache problems can be prevented—and pain lessened—if you learn how to sit and stand and move properly. (See chapter 6, Revitalize Your Spine.)

• If you stand for long periods, put one foot on a stool, alternating every few minutes. Prolonged standing fatigues the hip muscles and slowly pulls the pelvis forward. This causes a strain on the lower back muscles, which is relieved by lifting the foot slightly to return the spine to its natural curve.

• Sitting may be more stressful to your back than standing, since you lose the support of the pelvis when you sit down. If you have a bad back, don't cross your legs! It tilts the pelvis too far forward.

• Prop your feet up and sit with your knees level with or slightly higher than your hips.

• Two of the best-selling items at Boston's The Back Store are the Balans chair, which tilts slightly forward to relieve pressure on the lower back and transfer weight to the mid-thigh and a car-seat cushion that adjusts the spine to a more comfortable angle. Dr. Walpin has helped develop a contoured seat cushion (called "Bottoms Up" pelvic spinal posture aid) that supports the pelvis while limiting the harmful effects of gravity on the spine and pelvis. Those are just a few of the products available to take a load off your back.

• Some women find their backaches disappear miraculously when they take off their shoes. Others may not feel immediate pain when they wear high heels, but over a period of time, Dr. Walpin warns, high heels can cause slow, subtle damage to the back. "It's okay to wear shoes with heels up to an inch and a half," says Dr. Walpin.

• If you feel a back twinge coming on, lie on the floor, your head and buttocks supported by pillows and your legs resting on a chair. The trunk of your body should be moved as far under the chair as possible. This position will probably make you feel so good you may find yourself utilizing it again and again.

• Massage is nice anytime, but it's especially good when backache plagues your days and nights. Massage is a good way to work out a muscle spasm. It helps increase blood flow to the hurting areas and makes it relax.

• Stretch. Find yourself some good stretching exercises—even imitate a cat if you have to. Stretching enhances the flexibility of your back muscles and can give you momentary relief as well.

Muscle and Joint Aches

• Rest and exercise. It's as simple as that. You need to rest and relax a pained muscle or joint to ease the pain, and you need to exercise them to avoid stiffness and more pain. A regime of warm baths, massages and stretching exercises is good, according to Dr. Fries. He also recommends sponge-soled shoes for those who work on hard floors.

• If you do a lot of reading or needlework, place a fat, lightweight pillow across your lap. Not only will it support the weight of your arms, it will invite better posture and eliminate the chin-on-chest position.

• Wrap foam on the handles of tools you use often—even pens and pencils—to take the strain out of gripping. You can even use the foam cylinder from a curler.

Knee Pain

• Try "Baggie" therapy. That's the name coined by a group doctors at a Philadelphia hospital who found that bags of ice placed on arthritic knees for 20 minutes three times a day eased pain, gave sufferers more movement and strength, helped them sleep better and take less pain medication.

Leg Cramps

• They sneak up on you at night, an agonizing cramp in your leg (or foot) that seems to be ripping your muscle to shreds. Don't draw up your leg—stretch it. Get up and walk around, or massage or knead it like a lump of dough until it relaxes. A warm cloth also may help soften and calm the tensed muscle.

Menstrual Cramps

From the Federation of Feminist Women's Health Centers, come these tips:

• Relax, from head to toe. Lie back, resting your head on a pillow and elevate your legs over another. Concentrate on relaxing each set of muscles successively. Since the uterus is a muscle, you should find some relief from painful cramping.

• Try direct uterine massage. Press on the spot just above the pubic hairline where the uterus is located and gently massage.

• Have someone apply pressure to the lower back.

• Do the cobra exercise: Lie flat on the floor, gradually raising your head and chest without using your arms until your upper body is off the floor. Now, using your arms, raise your torso so your back is arched. Repeat several times until the lower back muscles relax.

Foot Pains

• For corns, cut plain moleskin into strips and place them on the corns to reduce the friction between your toes and shoes.

• Heal, hard, ugly calluses by soaking your feet for 15 minutes in warm water and applying moisturizer two or three times a day. Once they're soft, rub them with a pumice stone or another abrasive.

• For fallen arches, you should exercise, advises one podiatrist. Curl your toes, stretch your feel and rotate them to avoid the pain that radiates into your lower back.

• Massage sore feet with a foot roller or an empty soda bottle, gently rolling it back and forth with each foot several times a day.

• If your feet are stiff but not swollen, soak them in warm water for 15 minutes once or twice a day. If you have swelling, follow a 5-minute warm water soak with 2 minutes in cool water and repeat. Do this twice a day.

Burns

• Cold water usually relieves the pain of a minor burn. So does aloe vera. Use the fresh mucilaginous juice, applied directly from the plant leaf. Reapply as needed.

CHAPTER 5

Quit-Smoking Strategies That Really Work

Smokers are becoming an endangered species, but it's not just lung cancer or heart disease that's putting them there. Suddenly smokers are the new social outcasts. People shy away from them in restaurants, airplanes and buses. Corporations tuck them into little smoking rooms or forbid them to indulge at all on the job.

Without a doubt, antismoking sentiments are on the rise, and nowhere is that more evident than in California. Actually, if some Californians had their way, you'd have to go to Nevada to smoke. As it is, a number of cities and towns have passed the toughest no-smoking laws in the country. One community even forbids smoking in *all* public buildings.

But if California's laws are making it tough for smokers, they have at least one consolation—a successful and innovative antismoking program that's right in their own backyard. It's run by Carolyn Price, M.D., at the Smoker's Medical Clinic in San Francisco, and boasts an 80 to 85 percent success rate.

"Smoking is a medical addiction and can be as difficult to kick as heroin or alcohol," claims Dr. Price, who has worked with both drug and alcohol addicts in the past. "Many people claim to have stopped smoking, but they will not quit for good until they have conquered their nicotine withdrawal symptoms and found new behaviors to replace their smoking habits.

Because of its physiological, psychological and behavioral components, a good stop-smoking program must be multifaceted," she says. "At our clinic, the addiction problem is dealt with first.

"When a smoker inhales," explains Dr. Price, "the poisons put his system into shock. The body responds by putting out adrenaline in an attempt to speed up the chemical processes and rapidly eliminate the toxins. The smoker's blood flow, heart rate and blood pressure all increase so the smoker feels high for a while. It's interesting that the same energy which fights against the toxins has a side effect of giving you a feeling of well-being. But this is only temporary. As the body rids itself of nicotine, the heartbeat and other body processes slow down. The smoker feels relaxed for a while, then uncomfortable and a bit depressed. As blood sugar levels drop, he feels fatigued and tired. If another cigarette isn't smoked at this point, the smoker will begin to go through withdrawal and feel anxious and irritable."

Nicotine Neutralization Is the Key

Dr. Price counters these withdrawal symptoms with a technique called nicotine neutralization. If you've never heard of this treatment before, it's probably because it's practiced more in Europe than in the United States.

It's a technique not unlike acupuncture," says Dr. Price, "and takes specific training to learn." Specific points on the face and ears are injected with a local anesthetic and B vitamins. After the injections (which only need to be done once), the patient feels no psychological desire to smoke.

"We are uncertain why this technique works, but it does. It's most likely that the body's own natural painkillers—endorphins—are released. It may also interfere with IgE (a chemical in the body that affects allergies and the immune system).

Nevertheless, Dr. Price doesn't rely only on nicotine neutralization to help patients through the withdrawal phase. She also puts them on a special diet high in foods that will have an alkaline effect on the body. But, she warns, this should be done only under a doctor's supervision. "Foods such as beans, beet greens, raisins, spinach, carrots and many others cause the urine to become alkaline," explains Dr. Price. "And less than 1 percent of the nicotine is excreted when the urine is alkaline. Since the nicotine leaves the body so slowly, it drastically reduces the withdrawal symptoms."

By contrast, foods that make the urine acidic (beef, eggs and lentils are a few) cause the body to excrete four times as much nicotine as an alkaline diet.

"And I make sure that my patients are getting enough vitamins, especially C and B complex, for several reasons," she continues. "First of all, certain vitamins are depleted in smokers. Did you know that vitamin C is lost with each cigarette smoked? Vitamin A is reduced and

B's are lost too, and they're needed to counteract stress. What's more, vitamins C and E are excellent for detoxifying the body and may help decrease smoker's cough."

Still, it's important to remember that addiction is only one of the reasons people smoke, so nicotine neutralization is only *part* of the solution. The behavioral and psychological aspects must also be handled. "Do you know how many times a smoker lifts his hand to his mouth?" asks Dr. Price. "It's about eight times per cigarette, 160 times per pack. A heavy smoker may repeat this one movement over 300 times every day. And if they've been smoking for years, that behavior can really become embedded.

"So, if the patient feels very uncomfortable without a cigarette in his hand, I recommend SmokeBreak. This is a smokeless plastic cigarette that has the taste and smell of tobacco or menthol. It helps the patient recall the feelings associated with smoking and deal with the hand-to-mouth rituals."

To reduce the stress associated with quitting, Dr. Price teaches her patients relaxation techniques and deep-breathing exercises. They also take home a personalized tape recording of these lessons to assist them in the weeks following the procedure.

Try to Avoid Temptation

"For the social aspect, I tell my patients to stay away from cocktail parties or any other 'must smoke' situations for a while," she says. "Why tempt yourself?"

"I remember Dr. Price telling me that," says former patient Lucille Fjoslein, a San Francisco banker. "But I didn't listen. I'll never forget the day I quit. It was a bank holiday and I had my appointment with Dr. Price. I felt great when I left and headed straight to a pool party I had been invited to. I remember thinking that I didn't know what to do with my hands—but *I didn't want a cigarette!* I had no desire to light up.

"I had been smoking at least a pack and a half a day for many years and I had never been able to quit before. But I became a nonsmoker that day and haven't touched a cigarette since. It's been 1½ years now and I feel great."

"It was a piece of cake," adds Linda Sherwood of Palm Springs, California. "I never missed the smoking. Neither did my husband, Don. And we were your typical hard-core (three or four packs a day), down-to-the-filter smokers.

"Actually, at the time the procedure was being done, I thought, 'This has got to be a joke. It can't possibly work.' Yet right after the treatment, we drove from San Francisco to Palm Springs. That's eight hours in the car and we never wanted a cigarette.

"The best thing is that we started to feel better within a few days. I noticed the coughing diminished and I wasn't so short of breath. Now, after more than six months, I can even do aerobics and no more backing away."

"This is typical," Dr. Price told us. "Once a smoker quits, his body begins to return to normal. The cilia (microscopic hairs) in his lungs, which had ceased to function, begin sweeping out impurities again and precancerous lung cells gradually revert to normal. Then the better you feel physically, the easier quitting becomes."

Dr. Price's patients speak highly of the program and often recommend it to their friends who smoke. But the largest impact on Dr. Price's clinic has come from the no-smoking ordinances that have been passed. "These ordinances have brought up the smoking issue for discussion and debate, and that's good," says Dr. Price. "It's made people aware that health-oriented changes in the workplace can occur." And not just in California. Right now 38 states have passed smoking regulations. Fortunately, you don't have to go to California to get help to quit. There are programs all over the country that offer various techniques and support systems.

But first you have to want to quit. "Believe it or not, most people do want to," says Tracy Orleans, Ph.D., co-director, with Robert Shipley, Ph.D., of the Quit Smoking Clinic at Duke University Medical Center, in Durham, North Carolina. "In fact, 9 out of 10 have tried to quit or say they would if there were a viable way."

It Takes More Than Willpower

Dr. Orleans and Dr. Shipley use techniques that offer smokers a real chance at success. "You have to realize that quitting involves much more than willpower," says Dr. Orleans. "Even knowing the health risks isn't enough. Most already are aware of these risks but continue to smoke because they lack the skills and practical tactics to conquer the physiological addiction plus the psychological and behavioral dependencies. They also don't know that cigarette cravings and other withdrawal symptoms are only temporary, lasting only one or two weeks. It's not a life sentence of misery, even though at the time they're experiencing withdrawal it seems like it'll never end. So it's not surprising that the failure rate is highest between the seventh and tenth day.

"There are a number of scientifically tested techniques for helping people through withdrawal symptoms. We make use of a smoke-holding technique in our clinic sessions," says Dr. Orleans. "When the patient has a desire to smoke, we tell him to take a puff of the cigarette and hold the smoke in his mouth for 30 seconds. This is very unpleasant because it causes a bad taste in the mouth. The smoker then focuses on the negative sensations he is experiencing and sees himself not liking it.

"This is a type of aversive therapy that's highly effective and perfectly safe," Dr. Orleans continues. "I caution smokers against some other aversive techniques, however, particularly rapid smoking. The idea there is to smoke as fast as you can until it makes you violently nauseated and dizzy. This technique can be downright dangerous, especially for pregnant women or those with heart disease. Techniques involving rapid smoking do not appear to suppress smoking for more than a short time.

"Because smoke holding uses the natural properties of cigarette smoke, it has immediate and lasting beneficial effects. Best of all, this kind of technique has doubled clinic quit rates across the country."

Still, Dr. Orleans agrees with Dr. Price that overcoming withdrawal symptoms is only one aspect of the quit-smoking process. The behavioral and social conditioning that accompanies the smoking habit cannot be ignored, she stresses. "You've got to get away from cues—the little, sometimes unconscious signals that encourage you to light up. A cup of coffee after dinner, playing cards—stay away from the activities that tempt you the most.

"More important, though, is to find substitutes to take the place of those cigarettes," says Dr. Orleans. "Don't leave yourself empty-handed when the cravings occur. To keep hands busy, fiddle with paper clips or a Rubik's Cube. During a work break, read a magazine." Dr. Orleans also suggests that if you're hungry suck on cinnamon sticks, or munch on carrot sticks, or sugarless gum. Practice deep breathing and relaxation techniques when feeling stressed.

"Most smokers will see immediate benefits when they quit," says Dr. Orleans, "and this positive reinforcement helps get them through the toughest times. They'll be able to walk further without getting winded. Food will begin to taste better, too. They'll feel less anxious and more in control of their lives than when they smoked."

Even if better health is its own reward, don't shortchange yourself for a job well done. "Give yourself presents," says Dr. Orleans. "After all, you used smoking a cigarette as a kind of reward for a long time. Now with the money you're saving from not buying cigarettes you can substitute other rewards."

Rewards Can Be Incentives to Quit

Victor Strecher, Ph.D., of Temple University in Philadelphia, uses a reward system as an integral part of his no-smoking program. He developed his system for the Veterans Administration hospital in Ann Arbor, Michigan, to be used on the most incorrigible, long-term smokers. "These are the smokers that the doctors had given up on," says Dr. Strecher. "Even though many wanted to quit, they had no confidence they could do it."

Dr. Strecher and his staff worked to build the confidence of their patients by teaching them to recognize the cues that make them susceptible to the cigarette urge, how to develop substitutes and how to handle stress—much like Duke University Medical Center's program. The difference is that after the initial consultation, these patients were sent home with a self-help kit and did the rest on their own—with rewards for complying.

"The kit requires that each patient keep a dietary and answer questions about his progress. It also teaches them how to say no to a cigarette and how to avoid situations that induce smoking. Each week the patients had to send in the pages they had filled out. In return we would send them lottery tickets as their present.

"They loved getting those lottery tickets," Dr. Strecher says, "though we don't know if anyone actually won any money.

"But even more important is that these vets did it on their own. There wasn't a counselor to hold their hand every step of the way. I think this will improve their chances for long-term success, too, because it built up their confidence and made them believe in themselves."

"Our beliefs essentially determine our actions," adds John F. Balog, M.D., a Pasadena, California, psychiatrist who's known for his successful quit-smoking treatment. "In fact, because of my reputation for a high success rate, my patients automatically believe *they* will succeed, too."

Dr. Balog's technique is simplicity itself. "It's got to be easy or it won't work," he says. "It's a self-hypnosis method that can be learned in a few minutes and can be used anywhere. Here's how it works. First you roll your eyes upward, then close your eyes and breathe deeply. Take the index finger of your smoking hand and touch your cheek while you say the following words, 'I have a choice. I have the ability to quit smoking. I have power over my own life. I am responsible for my own health. I do not want to smoke anymore.'

"Saying those words during an altered state of consciousness helps you internalize them and *believe* in your ability to control your life," says Dr. Balog. This "trance" is a state of deep relaxation with increased focal attention and decreased outside awareness—like when you play a video game or become enthralled in a movie, explains Dr. Balog. "There's nothing mysterious about it."

But it does work—for about 60 percent of Dr. Balog's patients. "The power of suggestion is very strong. So strong, that it can overcome almost anything."

"The more you expect to succeed, the better your chances," adds Dr. Orleans. "But there's even a consolation for those who don't make it the first time. Don't give up. Studies show that the more you try to quit, the better your chances of eventually succeeding!"

What about Nicotine Gum?

You've probably seen or heard about nicotine gum by now if you're a smoker who's thought about quitting. It's been cleared for sale as a prescription drug by the Food and Drug Administration.

Chewing this gum is supposed to satisfy your nicotine cravings without the smoke. But if you think it will solve all your quit-smoking problems, you may be in for a disappointment. Not that the gum hasn't been shown to be effective. On the contrary, one British study showed that 47 percent of the people who participated in a smoking-cessation program aided by nicotine gum still weren't smoking a year later, compared to 21 percent in the placebo (blank) gum group (*British Medical Journal,* August 21, 1982).

But the gum can cause some unpleasant side effects, such as a lightheadedness and nausea—just as if you'd smoked a cigarette too rapidly. Other side effects include throat irritation, hiccups and excessive salivation. The experts also fear that patients will extract a prescription for the gum from their doctors without realizing that there's more to their habit than nicotine addiction. What's more, there's always the chance that these patients may simply be trading one bad habit for another.

Still, some doctors told us they would probably prescribe the gum for patients who wanted to try it, but only in conjunction with a behavioral counseling program—just the way the manufacturers of some nicotine gums recommend they be used.

CHAPTER 6

Revitalize Your Spine

Can you get out of a car in one seamless motion? Work in your garden without wondering how you are going to straighten up at the end of the day? Make love with no fear that your body is going to kink up in some weird position that only an emergency medical team can undo?

You can if your spine is strong and flexible, able to bounce back from the stress of daily life. If you can't, you can at least move in that direction by revitalizing the muscles, bone cartilage and nerves that make up your spine. How? With a program of careful exercise, nutrition and lifestyle changes.

• **Join an exercise class for people with back problems and stick with it.**

"Most back pains written off as disk problems are really muscle problems," says Willibald Nagler, M.D., New York Hospital/Cornell University Medical Center's physiatrist-in-chief. (A physiatrist is an M.D. specializing in physical medicine and rehabilitation.) "Most people with back problems have back and hamstring muscles too tight for toe touching, and abdominal muscles too weak for sit-ups."

The back and hamstring muscles support the entire structure of the back. They must be strong but flexible, to bend over, sit or twist without straining the back. The abdominal muscles, when strong, help to stabilize the lower back, the spine's most vulnerable point. Weak stomach muscles allow an exaggerated curve in the lower back, a posture that crimps disks and nerves.

To stretch the back and hamstring muscles, Dr. Nagler prescribes a series of exercises, including knee-to-chest pulls, cat curls and hip

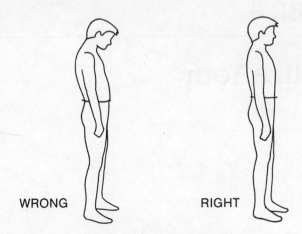

WRONG   RIGHT

Strengthening stomach muscles and stretching back muscles can help the correct the swayback posture typical in lower back pain.

rolls. To tighten the stomach, he recommends half sit-ups with knees bent, alternate leg lifts, pelvic tilts and other exercises. (An excellent program incorporating many of these exercises is "The Y's Way to a Healthy Back," offered at most YMCA's.) One word of warning: Rest, not exercise, is best when you are in true pain. And no excercise should hurt your back.

• **Assume the "S" Stance.** The trick to standing and walking is to find a posture that feels comfortable but offers your back maximum support. "We want to maintain the gentle 'S' curve of the spine," says Terry Nordstrom, director of the department of physical and occupational therapy and originator of the Back School of Stanford University. In the case of swayback, it helps to pull in the stomach and tuck under the buttocks. (See illustration above.) This tilts the pelvis toward the back and provides crucial support for the lower spine. Keep your knees slightly flexed, too. When you're standing a long time, you can tilt the pelvis back and flatten the small of your back by placing one foot on a stool, chair railing or other object a few inches high.

• **Sit Pretty.** Here again, you want to maintain the back's "S" curve. "People with lower back pain tend to flop into a chair or sofa, throwing their backs into a drooping "C" shape, says Edgar Wilson, M.D., a University of Colorado professor with a special interest in psychophysiology. This posture overstretches the lower back ligaments, while compressing the nerves passing out of the spinal column.

The easiest way to avoid slouching is to use a small pillow two or three inches thick behind your lower back when you sit. And avoid prolonged sitting. Take a stand-up break every hour.

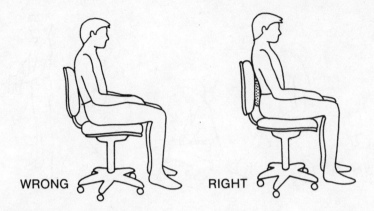

WRONG   RIGHT

Maintain the gentle "S" shape of your back when you sit by putting a small pillow behind your lower back.

• **Invest in a good chair.** Choose a chair that helps you to sit comfortably erect, not slumped forward. The ideal chair has a tiltable back support and adjustable height so you can sit with your feet flat on the floor and knees slightly lower or level with your hips. It has a contoured seat pan, not a square cushion, to help equalize pressure on the underside of your thighs, and (ideally) armrests to reduce stress getting in and out of the chair. (See illustration above.)

• **Don't drive yourself crazy.** If you're shopping for a new car, look for seats that offer good back support. Today many manufacturers are aware of the selling qualities of comfortable, supportive seating. Equip your older car with an orthopedic form. Keep the seat forward so your knees are raised to hip level; your right leg should not be fully extended.

• **Give your spine the nourishment it needs.** Osteoporosis and arthritis add to the back problems of many older people, especially women. Back pain can be a sign of microscopic fractures in the vertebrae, as the spine slowly crumbles from age-related calcium losses. Many bone specialists agree that, to prevent osteoporosis, most women should be getting at least 1,000 milligrams of calcium a day. That's about twice the current intake.

Vitamin D helps you absorb and use calcium. In one study, added vitamin D compound (calcitriol) reduced fractures in older women by 80 precent. If you're not drinking vitamin D-fortified milk or spending at least 15 minutes a day in the sun, consider taking a 400-International Unit vitamin D supplement daily.

Trace minerals like zinc, copper and manganese are also vital to

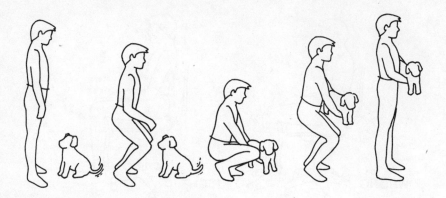

To lift, squat close to an object, bending your knees with your back straight and stomach muscles tensed. Then stand up slowly.

bone maintenance. Include shellfish, liver, nuts, seeds and whole grains in your diet to help meet these requirements.

Some researchers suggest vitamin C could help maintain spinal disks, because it helps form collagen, a tough connective tissue covering disks. Others have found that B complex also helps maintain bone and cartilage as well as soothe nerves irritated by rubbing vertebrae. And some doctors use supplemental magnesium to help relieve painful muscle spasms.

• **Check your footgear.** Any kind of pounding your feet take can show up as back pain, especially if your muscles are weak (strong muscles are good shock absorbers) or you're older (aging spinal disks become thin and hard, providing less cushioning for vertebrae). Switching to flexible-soled shoes with soft, shock-absorbing cushions produced significant pain relief in many patients treated in the orthopedics department of an Israeli hospital. The cushioning shoe inserts reduced—by 42 percent—incoming "shock waves" from pounding feet. Avoid heels higher than 1½ inches, which shift body weight forward and exaggerate swayback.

• **Visit a back store.** All kinds of goodies to pamper your back, including specially designed furniture and tools, positioning pillows, books and traction devices, can be found in a new kind of specialty shop—the back store. Check the phone book of the biggest city near you.

• **Learn to lift.** Never bend from the waist, even to pick up light objects, Nordstrom says. That deprives your spine of the support of the back muscles, which must relax to allow your body to flex. This places abnormal and uneven pressures on spinal disks. (See illustration above.)

• **Clean out your pocketbook.** An overweight pocketbook can do a number on your back, Nordstrom says. "We tell people to clean out their purses and briefcases, and to carry them as close to the body as possible. Over-the-shoulder is better than by hand." Try to keep your body from tilting with the weight of the object. And frequently switch the bag to the other shoulder. A backpack is a good alternative to the shoulder bag.

• **Drop your guard.** Relaxed muscles are less likely to go into painful spasms. "People who have been in pain for a while tend to tighten their muscles to guard the area, which makes it almost like a block of concrete," says Dr. Wilson.

Gentle stretching exercises, like yoga, are a good way to relax muscles. Biofeedback and progressive relaxation training can help you relax deeply, even while you're active.

• **Walk like a rag doll.** People with bad backs tend to walk ramrod stiff, Dr. Wilson says. "We have them walk as they imagine a Raggedy Ann doll would—floppy and leaning forward slightly, with knees slightly flexed, exaggerating the bouncy, relaxed walk we want them to develop."

• **Find your painless position.** "The key for anyone in acute pain is to rest in a neutral supportive position," says Nordstrom.

"You can lie on your back with several pillows under your legs and your knees somewhat bent. That reduces the stress on your back quite a bit and is usually most comfortable," Nordstrom says. "If you lie on your side, put a pillow or a small roll under your waist and a pillow between your legs. If you like lying on your stomach, put pillows under your belly to support your lower back."

• **Don't take it lying down.** Many people with aches and pains found that hard mattresses made them hurt more. Today, back experts recommend instead a bed that is level, with no sags, and firm enough to fully support the lower back.

A sheepskin or a soft inch-thick foam cover for your hard mattress may also help.

• **Sleep like a baby.** Sleeping positions make a big difference. Instead of lying on your back or stomach, sleeping in a fetal position is recommended. (See illustration on page 40.)

• **Seek the heat.** A warm bath or heating pad helps muscles relax. If you find yourself hunched into your blankets on chilly mornings, wear a turtleneck shirt to bed, Dr. Wilson suggests. When it's cold outdoors, keep your lower back warm with a jacket that covers your buttocks.

• **Lose that excess baggage.** Fat and back pain are an insepara-ble couple. "Especially when that weight is around their waist, people

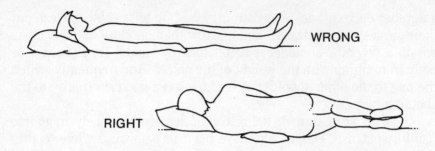

Lying flat on your back creates strain. Instead, curl into a fetal position and, if necessary, tuck a small pillow under your side.

are likely to have back problems," Nordstrom says. The weight greatly stresses soft back tissues and compresses disks. For maximum back protection and surest weight loss, combine diet with exercise.

• **Enroll in a back school.** Some hospitals, university medical centers and private physical-therapy clinics offer programs where you learn how to exercise, sit, stand, work and play in ways that help, rather than hurt, your back. Ask at the physical-therapy department of a local hospital for the location of the back school nearest you.

CHAPTER 7

25 Ways to Whip Your Allergies

Whoever said life isn't fair must have been thinking about allergies.

Some of us can plow through thickets of poison ivy and emerge without an itch. Others so much as brush up against a few spindly springs of the stuff, and they're digging holes through their pantyhose for weeks. For the majority of people, happiness is a warm puppy, yet dog fur brings thousands to heel. Why?

The reason is a difference in the sensitivity of the immune system. Burdened with an overprotective immune system, a person with allergies is forever on guard against everyday things that don't bother the rest of us. It might be a slice of fresh garden tomato or a patch of clover, a glass of milk or an affectionate kitten.

In most instances, allergies are more annoying than debilitating. Coping often involves avoiding foods to which you might be sensitive, or taking an antihistamine to dry up the occasional runny nose and soothe the itchy eyes of hay fever.

No matter what type of allergy you have, there's a good chance you can find relief. Here are 25 practical tips, based on current research and interviews with allergy experts.

1. Dietary Help for Migraines

Up to one-third of all migraines may be caused by food allergies, according to Lyndon E. Mansfield, M.D., clinical associate professor at Texas Tech University Health Sciences Center. The most common food "trigger" of migraines is wheat, followed by corn, peanuts and soybeans, with milk causing the most headaches in kids.

In some migraine sufferers, headaches start only after the patient has eaten a certain amount of offending food. In still others, stress—along with food—may trigger a migraine. But when these foods are avoided, Dr. Mansfield says, some people—not all—may have fewer headaches, less painful migraines or no headaches at all.

If your headaches have been diagnosed as migraines, consult an allergist for tests to discover possible food allergies.

2. Don't Pierce Young Ears

There's been an upsurge in allergic reactions to the metal nickel, particularly among girls under 15 who have had their ears pierced. In fact, nickel allergy is the most common contact allergy among women. The metal pins worn for the first three to six weeks after piercing contain minute quantities of nickel, which makes the body vulnerable to rashes later when metal comes into contact with skin. Reactions are common with jewelry, metal buttons, wristwatches, brassieres and eyeglass frames. Studies also show that girls with more than one hole in the ear—the "pin cushion" look—have twice as many allergies. Researchers recommend against ear piercing in children and young people.

3. Chew or Sip More Slowly

Sulfites are chemicals used to treat foods to make them look fresh. The Food and Drug Administration has banned the use of chemicals in supermarket produce or restaurant salad bars because they have induced fatal allergic reactions in people with asthma.

But we aren't rid of sulfites altogether. The FDA ban does not apply to prepared foods, such as potato products, frozen and canned vegetables, wine, beer, seafood, dried fruit, dry-mix salad dressings and soups. Even the most cautious person might not be able to avoid sulfites altogether.

But asthmatics, and others who could be allergic to sulfites, might be able to control an allergic reaction simply by eating or drinking more slowly. Up to 90 percent of all sulfite reactions are due to the release of sulfur dioxide gas from food when it is chewed and sipped according to Ronald Simon, M.D., a member of the FDA's advisory group on food additives. The allergic reaction is the result of inhaling sulfur dioxide. Many asthmatics have learned to drink and eat more slowly and watch for the warning signs of a reaction—itching, warmth, flushing, chest congestion, abdominal discomfort, coughing and wheezing.

4. Tell Your Dentist about Your Allergies

Nickel and sulfite allergies also surface in the dentist's office. Fillings, dentures, caps, braces and crowns may contain nickel. Local anesthetics may also be preserved with a sulfite chemical. If you're allergic to either substance, the dentist ought to be told before working in your mouth.

5. How to Avoid Eyeglass Rash

Spray polyurethane coating on eyeglass frames occasionally to avoid the itchy facial rash caused by the interaction of sweat with eyeglass materials.

6. Keep Kitty off the Bed

Cat got your nose? Could be it's been sleeping in your bed. Kitty's attachment to your bedcovers increases the amount of allergy-producing substances in your sleeping quarters a thousandfold. You don't have to hide your felines, though. Just keep them out of your bedroom. The same rule applies to Rover.

Additionally, if you can get your pets used to spending more time outdoors, you'll greatly reduce the amount of animal allergens—the microscopic particles that touch off your allergic reaction—in your house. Outdoors is also a good place to brush and pet your cat and dog.

7. Switch Sunscreen

If sunscreen on your shoulder makes you rashy, you might be allergic to PABA (para-amino benzoic acid).

PABA is not only precent in many commercial sunblocks, but in cosmetics as well. So it doesn't have to be summer for you to be affected.

To find out whether PABA turns your skin itchy and red, try a patch test first. Dab some PABA-containing lotion on a section of skin not normally exposed to the sun. Apply it two times a day for three days. If your skin doesn't break out, repeat the test on an exposed patch of flesh—the back of your hand is a good place. If you still don't react, you can probably use PABA without problems.

If you *do* react, try one of the many alternative sun screens such as benzophenone, sulsibenzone, oxybenzone, cinnamate compounds or the PABA derivative, octyl dimenthyl-PABA.

8. Squelch That Smoke

Cigarette smoke is bad enough, but for asthmatics, it could cause serious breathing difficulties. Second-hand cigarette smoke greatly increases the likelihood of an asthma attack for up to four hours, according to Australian researchers. Smoke evidently makes the asthmatic more sensitive to other allergens, like dust, cold air or exercise, they add.

43

Just leaving the smoke-filled room might not be enough. By the time you make your exit, it could be too late. To avoid the complications caused by smoke, you have to bypass the smoke altogether.

9. How to Have an Allergy-Free Baby

Oddly enough, some pregnant women crave foods to which they're allergic. If they don't get the food, they develop uncomfortable physical symptoms, like sweating and chills. Should you crave these foods during pregnancy, it might not be possible to avoid them altogether without some discomfort. But try to limit your intake and eat the desired food along with other foods, advises Vincent A. Marinkovich, M.D., a Stanford University pediatric allergist. Don't overdo any one food.

If you've already given birth to one child with a food allergy, he adds, avoid that food during the next pregnancy. Your next baby should be relatively free of food allergies.

10. Put the Squeeze on Your Asthma Inhaler

Asthmatics often use metered-dose inhalers to shoot a fine mist of medication into their bronchial tubes. But some people with arthritis or small hands have trouble squeezing the button atop the aerosol bottle. Others just have trouble coordinating the effort, pushing down on the top of the bottle and inhaling at the same time.

Glaxo, Inc., has developed a plastic squeeze trigger, called VentEase, that slips over the inhaler to make it easier to use. To get one free, ask your doctor or pharmacist, or call Glaxo's medical department at 800-334-0089.

11. Sniff for the Hidden Scent

Cosmetic and grooming-aid manufacturers sell a lot of products marked "unscented." But the fragrance may actually be masked with a chemical, ethylene brassalate. If you're allergic to fragrances, beware. Doctors believe you can react to this neutral scent just as easily as you might to any other fragrance. Read the label, and avoid ethylene brassalate.

12. Close Your Air-Conditioner Vent

An air conditioner can do a lot of good for a person allergic to pollen or fungus spores. But if you keep the vent control in the open position, you're sucking outside air—and pollen—indoors. Pollen is extremely small, so your air-conditioner filter probably can't screen it all out. Also, research shows that often there is a brief "burst" of mold contamination when the air conditioner is turned on because of mold inside the machine. So turn on the air conditioner and leave the room for half an hour.

Some people are very sensitive to cold air. So if your air-conditioner temperature control is set to "cold," turn it up to around 70 degrees.

Automobile air conditioners are subject to the same hazards, so keep the vent closed, and run the air conditioner with the car windows open for a few minutes before you get in. And keep the temperature temperate.

13. Ragweed Sufferers Might Be Ripe for Melon Allergy

Some people who are allergic to ragweed also develop itching or swelling of the lips, tongue or throat after eating watermelon, cantaloupe, honeydew, zucchini or cucumber. According to the Allergy Research Laboratory of Detroit's Henry Ford Hospital, these fruits and vegetables have allergy-producing proteins almost identical to those found in ragweed.

14. Avoid Fur-Bearin' Varmints

If you're allergic to cats and dogs, it's likely you'll also react where the deer and the antelope play. If you're a hunter, that means getting someone else to handle animal carcasses. If you're a "hunter's widow," don't handle your husband's hunting clothes.

15. Go Easy on Shellfish If You're Allergic to Shrimp

Chances are pretty good you're also allergic to crayfish, lobster, clams, oysters and crab, according to physicians from the clinical immunology section at Tulane University Medical Center. Common reactions include hives, nausea and shortness of breath.

16. Declare War on Dust Bunnies

Many people are allergic to substances found within their own homes, particularly dust. But you can keep dust down by doing any one of the following things:

Have a contractor clean out your heating system. All it takes is a couple of carbon-dioxide fire extinguishers and just a little time.

If you're redoing an allergy-sufferer's room, forget rugs. Instead, use linoleum in solid sheets, not blocks. Mold hangs out in the cracks between linoleum blocks.

If you're wallpapering, purchase mold-free paper paste. If you're painting, have mold preventive added to the paint.

Finally, when you plaster, look for the one-coat variety that doesn't need sanding.

17. Try This New Test for Children's Food Allergies

It's called a MAST test, and it's a great improvement over the uncomfortable standard method of testing for allergies, which involves placing tiny food samples under the child's skin and waiting for a reaction.

For the MAST test, all the doctor needs is a small blood sample, according to Dr. Marinkovich. The MAST test uses a small chamber divided into sections, each of which contains a thread coated with a specific allergen. After blood is placed in the chamber, the doctor examines the threads to determine whether antibodies in the blood are reacting to the allergens.

The MAST procedure can detect allergic reactions to 35 different foods. The test is particularly accurate in pinning down children's food allergies. In adults it is less accurate because their circulating antibodies are different.

18. Stick to White Glue

Many of the advanced "super" adhesives do dry more quickly and hold better, but some people who use them develop other allergic reactions, such as asthma.

19. Be Satisfied with Not-So-Soft Sheets

Some of the laundry-softener strips cause allergic reactions. For most of us, that may not be a problem, but if you develop a chronic runny nose, coughing, wheezing, asthma or skin rash, fabric-softener sheets might be the cause. One manufacturer has investigated 300 such complaints.

20. Consider an Air Cleaner

Newer models are very effective at removing dust, pollen, cigarette smoke and mold from the household environment. Cheap models are considerably less effective, according to Harold S. Nelson, M.D., chairman of the American Academy of Allergy and Immunology's Committee on Environmental Controls.

Since an air cleaner can be expensive, Dr. Nelson recommends leasing one first to see if it does the job. Take time to decide whether it moves enough air, and try it out in your bedroom a couple of nights to find out how much noise it makes. When you use an air cleaner, put it in the middle of the room, where it can do the most good.

21. The Solution to Contact-Lens Contact Allergies

If you wear contacts and get itchy, teary or swollen eyes, it could be an allergic reaction to thimersol, a mercury preservative used in contact-lens solutions. Another common ingredient, the enzyme papain, can also cause allergic reactions. Switch to solutions that contain neither.

22. Shield Yourself Against Poison Oak and Ivy

A new product, Ivy Block, appears to prevent the sap from these plants from irritating the skin. The aerosol spray has undergone testing with forest firefighters in California, with reported success. The spray isn't available over the counter yet, but it is being offered through dermatologists and allergists. Ask about it if poison ivy or oak make you itchy.

If you don't have such a product, and you find yourself exposed to either poison plant, here's what to do, according to William Epstein, M.D., professor of dermatology at the University of California at San Francisco. Wash the affected area immediately with rubbing alcohol, followed by water, and wash everything you might have touched with water. And don't use a washcloth, since this will also pick up and spread the poison.

23. Yes, You *Can* Garden

All you have to do is observe a few precautions.

Do your gardening in the evening. Most weeds unleash their pollen in the morning. Also, water the soil regularly to keep the dust and molds down, and wear gardening gloves if you have sensitive skin.

24. How to Survive a Pointed Encounter with a Stinging Insect

It's hard to believe a tiny insect can do so much damage, but an allergic reaction can lead to anaphylactic shock, which is life threatening.

If you are sensitive to insect stings, immunotherapy can help. This involves being injected every few weeks with gradually increasing quantities of diluted venom. But just because it's November and all the bees and wasps are asleep doesn't mean you should stop getting your shots, says Martin D. Valentine, M.D., a professor of medicine at Johns Hopkins University School of Medicine. If you stop during the winter you'll lose the protection you've built up.

25. Here's More Insect Protection

If you can avoid being stung in the first place, you can avoid a possible allergic reaction. Here are some ideas:

Wear sandals instead of going barefoot. Most stings happen when people tiptoe barefoot through the tulips.

Also, check woodpiles for nests before you stack logs on top. In warmer weather, the same goes for picnic tables.

Finally, gently shake an opened beverage can before putting it to your lips. If you hear buzzing inside, there's probably something alive in there.

CHAPTER 8

Keeping Indigestion
Out of Your Life

According to Mariam Ratner, associate director of the American Digestive Disease Society, 50 percent of all Americans suffer from occasional digestive distress. And, apparently, most of them are running to the pharmacy for something—anything—to calm their gastrointestinal storm. By one estimate, the yearly bill for nonprescription digestion soothers amounts to 25 percent of all over-the-counter drug sales, about $1.25 billion.

You can blame indigestion for most of this digestive disarray. But do you have to put up with it? Probably not. And you can usually treat it without adding to over-the-counter drug sales.

A Burning Inside

Take heartburn, for example. "The real cause of heartburn—this hot sensation under the breastbone—is what we call esophagus reflux," says Gordon McHardy, M.D., emeritus professor of medicine at Louisiana State University Medical Center. "The esophagus, of course, is the tube that carries the food from your mouth to your stomach At its lower end, there's a muscle that relaxes to let food into your stomach, then immediately contracts to close off the esophagus from the stomach contents. If the muscle fails, acid and bile from the stomach can back up into the unprotected esophagus and irritate it. And it's this irritating backwash, or reflux, that causes the burning sensation in the chest."

The burning in the chest is frequently mistaken for a heart attack. Or worse—heart attacks are often labeled heartburn.

"The burning sensation can often turn into actual pain," says Dr.

McHardy. "And the pain can mimic that of a heart attack by radiating into the neck and left shoulder. In fact, most people who experience such severe heartburn for the first time go to a hospital emergency room or to their physician."

And so they should. Some gastroenterologists say that if you aren't absolutely sure what that burning pain means, you should call your doctor.

Chronic heartburn can sometimes lead to heavy-duty medical troubles. Myron D. Goldberg, M.D., a New York City gastroenterologist and author of *The Inside Tract: The Complete Guide to Digestive Disorders* (Beaufort Books), says, "Millions of people suffer from the symptoms without suffering any ill effects, except, of course, for the discomfort of the symptoms themselves. But, and this is very important, if a chronic [reflux] esophagitis is not treated properly, it can develop into a more serious problem. The constant back flow of acid can cause ulcers in the esophagus, because the delicate tissues there are susceptible to damage by stomach acid and even bile. This can lead to scarring of the esophagus and eventual narrowing, which can make swallowing food difficult or even impossible."

So what can you do about the gastric fire? Some people down a glass of warm milk to cool the flames. Some try peppermint to dull the pain. A few do their best to belch the burn away. But these "curatives" are just more heartburn lore—and are completely worthless. In fact, gastric experts claim that these remedies can actually make symptoms worse. Milk can stimulate stomach acid secretion. And acid, of course, is part of the problem. Peppermint is one of several substances that can weaken the muscle that opens and closes the esophagus's trapdoor. And belching can bring acid up into the esophagus lining.

As you would expect, the only real cures or preventives are those that reduce the chances of bile or acid splashing into the tender esophagus. And there's plenty of agreement among gastric physicians on how to do that:

• Avoid the substances that weaken or relax that critical esophagus muscle—caffeine, alcohol, chocolate, peppermint, even decaffeinated coffee. Research has implicated cigarette smoking, too.

• If you're overweight, take off some pounds. Says Dr. Goldberg, "Excess weight increases intra-abdominal pressure, which aggravates the reflux process."

• Shrink your meals and reduce their fat content. "Over-eating distends the stomach," says Dr. McHardy. "And distension strains the esophagus muscle. Fatty meals can do the same thing because the stomach takes longer to digest them, and that can only distend the stomach longer."

• Put gravity to work for you. When the pain hits, don't lie down unless you have to. Stand up and loosen all tight clothing to let gravity force your stomach acid downward and away from your esophagus. The same principle applies while sleeping. By hiking the head of your bed up on six-inch blocks, you can often ease your symptoms or stop them before they start. Propping yourself up with pillows, though, is *not* a good variation on this technique. Propping means bending, which puts pressure on that esophageal gatekeeper.

• Try a simple remedy: water. "Believe it or not," says Dr. Goldberg, "water works very well. If you drink a glass of cold water, it will wash the acid from the surface of the esophagus back into your stomach."

• Exercise moderately. According to some gastroenterologists, exercise doesn't contribute to heartburn—it may actually help prevent it. "Vigorous exercise, such as weight lifting, may strain the abdomen and may readily contribute to reflux into the esophagus," says Dr. McHardy. "But moderate exercise—like walking, for example—can be beneficial."

Then, of course, you need to avoid those things that raise your stomach's acid level. Obviously, too much acid can worsen heartburn. Not to mention an "acid stomach." That's another brand of gastric fire, a burning sensation in the stomach itself.

Most people know that certain foods can either boost the stomach's production of acid or add extra acid to the stomach's own mix. What they don't always understand is which foods actually are the worst offenders: milk, onions, peppers, mustard, horseradish, coffee, alcohol, curry, orange juice, aspirin and tomato juice.

Scientists have known for decades that tension, anger and anxiety can trigger the release of stomach acid. So eating a meal when you're steamed or strained is a known formula for gastric distress. As soon as the food reaches your stomach, hydrochloric acid oozes from the stomach wall. Other gastric juices join in and digestion proceeds. Tension trips a signal and even more acid pours in. The mucosa, the tough lining of the stomach, is designed to withstand the acidic concoction that your stomach pumps out. But you can still feel the gastric burning that the excess acidity brings on.

"Some people have a normal tendency to secrete more acid," Dr. McHardy says. "And some simply enhance acidity through questionable habits."

The Pain of Intestinal Gas

What about the annoying—and often painful—affliction known as gas. Eating the wrong foods is one cause. But a surprising amount of gaseous distress is actually caused by what doctors call aerophagia—swallowing air. Food itself contains a lot of air. An apple, for example, is 20 percent air.

But certain eating habits—usually brought on by nervousness—draw in more air than we can easily expel. "Some people swallow excessive amounts of air without even realizing it," says Albert I. Mendeloff, M.D., chief of research medicine at Sinai Hospital of Baltimore. "They eat too fast, gulp down their food, suck on hard candy, chew gum and sigh repeatedly. They may take in 100 milliliters of air and belch out only 90, which leaves an excess. After a while the surpluses mount up, often causing a lot of discomfort."

The extra air collects mostly in the stomach—sometimes in a single giant bubble called a magenblase—and simply won't go away. A good belch may not help. You may, like some people, swallow air just before you force a belch. And that would put you right back where you started. Avoiding the habits and foods that caused the problem in the first place generally prevents it.

The other gas—the more painful and embarrassing kind—doesn't have much to do with swallowed air. "Most of the gas that is passed rectally," says Dr. Goldberg, "comes from the activity of the normal intestinal flora upon undigested foodstuffs."

And as you probably know, some foods undergoing that process produce more gas than others. For people with lactose intolerance, milk products are among the worst offenders. And for most everyone, certain fiber foods can be gas makers, too—beans, celery, broccoli, raisins, cauliflower, carrots, cabbage and others.

That shouldn't stop you, however, from getting the fiber your body needs. "How much fiber you should eat depends on how well your system handles it," says Dr. Goldberg. "Each person has to find his or her own middle ground by trial and error," he says. "What may seem to be an excessive amount of fiber for one person is a perfectly acceptable amount for another."

Besides, your body has a way of adjusting over time to gas-making fiber foods. Says Dr. Goldberg, "The intestinal bacterial flora may adapt in such a way that these foods become less gaseous with their continued use." At any rate, for gas of the gut there's a highly regarded remedy: exercise. "Walking, climbing stairs, riding a bicycle—these may help when nothing else will," says Dr. Mendeloff.

CHAPTER 9

Solve Your Foot and Heel Problems Now

With all the new information that's available about the care and maintenance of the human foot, there's really no reason for you to put up with foot pain anymore. The same walking and jogging boom that introduced thousands of American soles to blisters and sore arches also mothered the invention of lots of useful foot-saving shoes and devices and exercises.

If you want to understand how to solve your foot problems, you should first understand what happens to your feet during locomotion.

Active people tend to develop foot pain in two places. One of them is the heel. When you jog or run, your heels hit the ground with a force greater than your weight. The heel of a 150-pound jogger, it's been estimated, hits the ground with a force of 255 pounds, and the heel of a runner of the same weight hits the ground with a force of roughly 375 pounds—over and over and over.

Couple those statistics with the fact that the layer of fat globules that cushioned our heels during youth becomes thinner and less resilient with age, and it's not surprising that heel pain strikes many an adult jogger.

The other area of trouble is the arch, and its problem has a fancy name: plantar fasciitis, or inflammation of the plantar fascia. The plantar fascia is a tough band of fibrous tissue that crosses the sole, linking the heel bone to the ball of the foot. With every step we take, all our weight comes down on the fascia, pushing the arch down and in. In an exercise program of walking or running, excessive pronation (rolling in of the foot) causes more rapid pulling of the fascia from the bone.

53

Why Your Heel May Hurt . . .

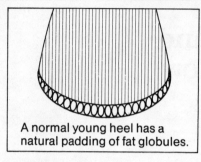

A normal young heel has a natural padding of fat globules.

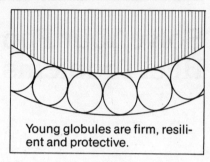

Young globules are firm, resilient and protective.

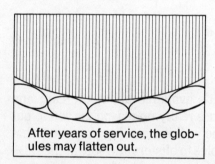

After years of service, the globules may flatten out.

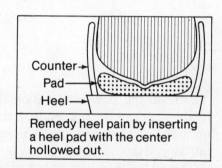

Remedy heel pain by inserting a heel pad with the center hollowed out.

In time, the fascia may stretch and become inflamed. It may even begin to tear away from the heel bone, causing the formation of a bony growth called a heel spur. Heel spurs themselves are seldom painful, but the increased pulling of the tissue away from the bone that often accompanies fasciitis is the most common source of foot pain among adults who exercise.

"A good percentage of the walking or jogging population has symptomless heel spurs to some extent," says Phillip Perlman, D.P.M., a Boulder, Colorado, podiatrist who specializes in runners' foot problems. "Jogging or running may speed up the separation process, thus producing painful symptoms."

"People can usually diagnose themselves," says Dr. Perlman, who often jogs with his patients to observe their form. "It's fasciitis if it feels like a stone bruise on the heel that won't go away, or if there's pain as soon as you roll out of bed in the morning."

Dr. Perlman advises against x-rays. "X-rays are expensive, the body doesn't need the radiation exposure, and most of the time they aren't necessary," he says. Some podiatrists use injections of cortisone into the heel to stop the inflammation and pain, or perform surgery to separate the fascia from the heel bone. Dr. Perlman uses these options only when all else fails.

Freeze the Pain

Ordinary ice may be the best treatment for fasciitis. One thing Dr. Perlman sometimes suggests to his patients is to put on two pairs of socks and then slip some ice between the two layers. Keep the ice there for about 20 minutes, he says, and repeat the process three to five times a day until the pain subsides. An alternative: John Grady, D.P.M., of Chicago, tells his patients to fill a Styrofoam cup full of water, freeze it, then strip away the edge of the cup and massage the painful area with this cylindrical icicle as needed. Applying ice right after a workout seems to help many runners.

In his book *Foot and Ankle Pain* (F. A. Davis), Rene Cailliet, M.D., of the University of California School of Medicine, says that both gentle heat or cold can help any sort of foot strain. Try cold first, then heat, he says, or alternate a cold foot bath with a warm one.

Many people try to prevent or cure their foot problems by shopping for an arch support or heel cushion that they can slip into their shoes. If this doesn't do the trick, then a professional orthotic may work better. An orthotic is an arch and heel support custom made from a plaster cast of your foot. Orthotics can cost as much as $300, however, and most people look for something "off the rack" and less costly.

There are several kinds of inexpensive insoles designed to absorb the shock of walking and running. Scholl manufactures a green foam pad called Pro Comfort, as well as arch supports. Spenco makes a whole family of insoles and arch supports. Insoles made from a super-resilient material called Sorbothane are also popular, although some people say they're too heavy. These products are available in sporting-goods stores and running-shoe stores.

Many foot-pain sufferers go searching for the ideal jogging shoe for their feet. Since running shoes are expensive—up to $85 for one model—you might want to consult a sports-minded podiatrist before laying your money down.

There's also a new breed of shoes on the market that combines the handsome leather uppers of a street or casual shoe with the cushioning, light weight and rugged sole of a jogging shoe. The Rockport Company of Massachusetts offers a line of smart walking shoes called RocSports. The Danner Shoe Company of Oregon makes a sturdy shoe called

When Your Achilles Tendon Is A-Killing You

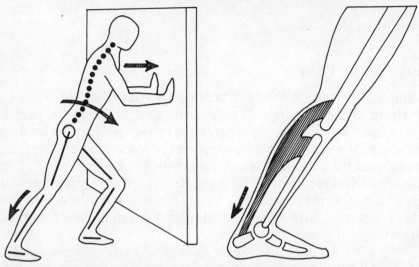

This exercise relieves heel pain by stretching the Achilles tendon. Keep rear heel on the ground and rear leg straight. With palms on the wall, flex the forward leg at the knee and lean forward as though you were pushing a stalled car. Do this with each leg.

Danner Urban Lights. Podiatrists may recommend these shoes for salespeople, nurses, letter carriers and anybody else who stands or walks for a living.

For blisters, two veteran walkers we know recommend Second Skin, made by Spenco. Second Skin is a small piece of transparent film that's premoistened. It's designed to clean the wound, protect it from friction and hold moisture in. Moleskin, a Scholl product, also seems to help blisters. Moleskin is cloth with an adhesive backing. Some people apply it in advance to prevent blisters wherever they usually get them. Ordinary white adhesive tape may also help.

A product called Johnson's Foot Soap comes highly recommended for the aches and pains of a walker's feet. On the market since 1870, Johnson's Foot Soap contains soap flakes, borax, iodine and bran. Mix one of the individual packages in two quarts of water, then soak your feet. It helps promote circulation and softens the tough outer layer of the foot.

Keep On the Grass

Whirlpool baths can also soothe aching feet. Many mail carriers say that after beating the pavement all day, they sometimes head for the whirlpool at their local athletic club. A number of companies, including Clairol and Pollenex, manufacture small household foot baths for between $30 and $80.

You can help your feet considerably by walking or jogging on grass instead of concrete. One podiatrist says that farmers, above all others, retain good foot structure throughout their lives because they spend so little time on hard pavement.

If you are overweight, losing weight might be the best way to take a load off your feet, podiatrists say. Also, arthritis, gout or diabetes could cause foot pain. Arthritis twists the bones out of shape, causing considerable pain when you walk. Gout is caused by the deposit of uric acid crystals at the joints. And diabetes, which prevents good circulation at the extremities, is another possibility. All three of these conditions require a doctor's attention.

Ultimately, there's more at stake in the treatment of foot pain than just the comfort of your feet. The posture of our feet influences the bone structure of the whole body, and the health of the whole body often relies on the exercise we get while walking or running. Our feet, and how we care for them, can make all the difference.

Flexing the Feet

Certain exercises can help get you back on your feet if you've been laid up by foot pain. Here's one of them:

Slip off your shoes and sit with your feet dangling above the floor. With lots of energy, point your toes down, then in, then up, and then out, so that you make circles in the air with your big toes. Simultaneously flex and extend your toes. Dr. Cailliet says these exercises strengthen your leg and foot muscles.

Here are a few exercises you can do while standing:

Place your feet apart and pointing in, as if you're a little pigeon-toed. Roll onto the outside of your feet several times, and curl your toes tightly. Also, practice walking on your toes, slightly pigeon-toed. When you're walking to lunch or in the shopping mall, it also helps to purposely put some bounce into your stride.

CHAPTER 10

A Health Guide to the Breasts

Finding a lump in your breast can be frightening. Even when it's happily resolved with the diagnosis of "benign," the experience can leave you feeling vulnerable about this part of your body, wondering what you can do to avoid being a victim of chronic breast pain, or worse, the 1 in 11 women who gets breast cancer.

Knowing about your breasts—how they function and their disorders—is a good way to minimize that feeling of vulnerability.

Breasts are made up of fat, honeycombed with milk-producing glands and ducts that respond to changes in body chemistry. The milk-producing cells lining the glands are controlled cyclically by three major female hormones—estrogen, progesterone and prolactin. In a woman of childbearing age, each month these cells are stimulated to grow and to accumulate fluids. This makes many woman's breasts feel heavy, and sometimes painful and lumpy, three or four days before their period. When menstruation begins, this hormonal stimulation stops. In a healthy breast, cell growth and fluids subside and pain disappears.

In some women, though, premenstrual pain is severe or becomes a month-long problem. Why this happens is something researchers are still figuring out. It's most likely related to imbalance in hormone levels—too much estrogen or too little progesterone, says Robinson Baker, M.D., director of the Breast Clinic at Johns Hopkins Hospital in Baltimore. And it may be influenced by other body chemicals produced by stress or stimulated by certain foods.

Lumpy, painful breasts are one of many ailments that doctors place in the catchall category "fibrocystic disease."

"Most doctors will agree that lumpy, painful breasts are perfectly normal," says Susan M. Love, M.D., clinical instructor in surgery at Harvard Medical School. "Sixty percent of women have breasts painful enough to go to the doctor sometime during their lives. Not because they want relief from the pain but because they're worried that they have cancer. If you can reassure them that this is okay and that they do not need treatment, most are perfectly happy."

Other doctors *do* agree that painful, lumpy breasts are common. But, as we'll see later, they don't all agree that the condition is normal or necessarily healthy.

More severe forms of fibrocystic disease involve three separate types of breast conditions—fibrosis, the formation of cysts, and changes in the cells lining the milk ducts, says Dr. Baker.

In fibrosis, the connective tissue that supports the milk ducts grows and thickens into scar tissue, perhaps as a result of too much estrogen, Dr. Baker says. In itself, fibrosis is not painful. But frequently it is accompanied by the formation of cysts. The milk ducts, blocked by tissue growth, are unable to drain properly and swell up into tender, fluid-filled sacs. Cysts can range in size from barely palpable to large enough to hold more than a quarter of a cup of water, and they can form in a week or two, Dr. Baker says.

Small cysts often shrink on their own; larger cysts are often punctured and drained with a needle. If they recur several times in the same spot, they may be removed surgically.

Most doctors now say fibrocystic disease in itself does not lead to breast cancer—that is, cysts do not become cancerous. Sometimes, though, some forms of this disease include overgrowth and abnormalities in the cells lining the milk ducts. This condition, known as proliferative, or hyperplastic, disease, can develop into a malignancy, although only a small number do, Dr. Baker says. The only way to diagnose this condition is by tissue biopsy.

All women, whether they are at risk for cancer or not, should examine their breasts each month. For a woman with fibrocystic disease, though, the question is how to distinguish all those lumps and bumps from one that might actually be cancerous. This is where regular breast self-exams become important. The idea is to become so familiar with your breasts, lumps and all, that when you find something different or unusual, you recognize it for what it is and have it checked out. "Any discrete mass should be biopsied, regardless of a patient's age," Dr. Baker says. But there *are* ways to distinguish between benign and malignant lumps.

A cyst will be tender and move easily. It feels similar to an eyeball felt through an eyelid. A cancerous lump is often painless. It will seem to be anchored to the chest wall or to the breast tissue. Cysts can occur in both breasts simultaneously, but cancer usually occurs in one breast only, most often in the upper-right quarter nearest the shoulder.

Your own greatest risks for developing breast cancer are, unfortunately, things you cannot control. If your mother, sister or grandmother developed breast cancer, your own chances of getting it are two to three times greater than the general population. If the cancer developed prior to menopause or was in both breasts, the risk is even higher. If you've already had cancer in one breast, your chances of getting it in the other breast are five times greater than if you'd never had cancer.

Breast cancer is unusual in women under age 30. Its incidence begins to rise in the early 40's, but it's still relatively uncommon up to age 50. Most breast cancers are found in women ages 55 to 60.

There are ways, though, to decrease your odds, both for bothersome but benign breast ailments and breast cancer. More and more, prevention-minded health professionals are observing, and researchers are confiming, that breast disease is influenced by one factor we can do something about—our diet.

Keeping Your Breasts Healthy

"I believe in taking a broad approach," says Phyllis Havens, a registered dietician with the Holistic Center in South Portland, Maine, who counsels many women with breast tenderness and swelling and other premenstrual symptoms. "I recommend some major dietary changes and vitamin supplementation."

These include eliminating caffeine-containing foods and fat-rich dairy products, cutting back on red meats, sugars and fats, and adding safflower oil, fiber-rich vegetables and vitamins E and B complex.

Havens's and others' observations that this sort of diet relieves breast disease and problems with other estrogen-sensitive tissues like the uterus and ovaries, is being confirmed, at least in part, by laboratory research.

John Minton, M.D., Ph.D., of the department of surgery, Ohio State University College of Medicine in Columbus, has found that substances contained in certain foods can aggravate breast symptoms. These substances produce biochemical signals that activate enzymes that promote fibrous tissue and cyst fluid development in women with fibrocystic disease.

"I know that most women can reverse lumpy, painful breasts completely with changes in their diet," he says.

Dr. Minton discovered that eliminating foods containing substances called methylxanthines (which include caffeine and are found in coffee, tea, cola and chocolate) was associated with the disappearance of breast cysts in most women within a few months.

But he also noted that some women who initially got much better on the diet later got worse.

"We discovered that when they stopped drinking coffee, they were somehow attracted to other foods that were giving them the same biochemical kick," Dr. Minton says. They include some dairy products, particularly cheese.

Christiane Northrup, M.D., a South Portland, Maine, gynecologist who refers some of her patients to the Holistic Center for nutritional counseling, prescribes 800 to 1,200 International Units (I.U.) daily of vitamin E for her patients with fibrocystic disease. "I find it helps a great deal to relieve pain and swelling, especially when the symptoms occur because of rapidly changing hormone levels that come with menopause," she says. (This level of supplementation should only be used with your doctor's approval and supervision.)

Preliminary research by Robert Dondon, M.D., director of reproductive medicine at North Charles General Hospital in Baltimore, suggests that vitamin E may be of value in treating breast cysts. In one study, 80 percent of the women responded to 600 I.U. of vitamin E daily for two months with decreased symptoms of pain. His current work does not indicate that vitamin E lowers levels of estrogen or progesterone.

Can Vitamin A Help?

What about vitamin A? Can this apparent cancer inhibitor protect against breast disease? The answers aren't in yet, but there's a tremendous amount of interest in its possible use, says Marc Lippman, M.D., director of the National Institutes of Health Breast Cancer Division.

"The data from animal studies is quite encouraging," Dr. Lippman says. "Forms of vitamin A can prevent the action of some tumor promoters, there's no doubt about it." In tissue cultures, vitamin A prevents the proliferation, or uncontrolled growth, of breast tissue cells.

One of the most promising forms of vitamin A for breast cancer, based on work done by Richard Moon, Ph.D., is a retinoid called 4-hydroxyphenylretinamide, which was surprisingly effective in preventing breast tumors in mice exposed to carcinogens, says Frank Meyskens, M.D., associate professor in the department of medicine at the University of Arizona, Tucson.

Maurice Black, M.D., of the Institute for Breast Disease of the New York Medical College, is using short-term high oral doses of both vitamins A and E in women who have had one breast cancer. This study arose as an offshoot of an ongoing investigation of the protective effect of specific cell-mediated immunity against the patient's own tumor. In the course of these studies patients were identified who lacked this immunity. It was those nonreactive patients who participated in the high-dose vitamin studies.

These women don't naturally show the kind of immune response associated with good survival rates, Dr. Black says. But with large doses of either A or E, 50 to 60 percent do show this immune response; and with both A and E, 80 percent show the response, Dr. Black says. "We don't yet know if this induced response works as well as a spontaneous response. We haven't been following these women long enough to see if they have a reduced incidence of recurrent and/or second primary breast cancer." (Large doses of vitamin A shouldn't be taken without medical guidance.)

Selenium Shows Promise

Selenium seems to have a protective effect. "The results of animal and human population studies continue to be encouraging that the risk of breast cancer does decline if selenium intakes are high," says Gerhard Schrauzer, Ph.D., professor of chemistry at the University of California at San Diego. In mice bred to carry a virus which puts them at high risk of developing breast cancer, those receiving extra selenium had an incidence of breast tumors that was 10 percent lower than those that received no additional selenium. "And there's increasing evidence that many human breast cancers have a similar viral influence," Dr. Schrauzer says. Mice fed a high-fat diet and exposed to cancer-causing chemicals also had fewer, slower-forming tumors with selenium supplementation.

"Human studies with selenium and breast cancer have yet to be done on a large scale, but ongoing studies in Finland and Australia with women with benign fibrocystic disease are showing that selenium supplementation does seem to have beneficial effects," Dr. Schrauzer says. This is a hopeful sign that this unpleasant condition will, in the future, become preventable and treatable by nutritional means. Foods high in selenium include seafoods, liver, kidneys, meat and some whole grains. Supplements of more than 100 micrograms shouldn't be taken.

Cut Back on Fat

Your best bet against both benign breast disease and breast cancer may be the same thing that helps protect against heart disease—a low-fat diet. Population studies show a strong parallel between fat consumption and the incidence of breast cancer. Countries with low-fat diets like Japan and Thailand have only about one-quarter the number of breast cancer deaths as the United States, Denmark, and the Netherlands, where people consume up to twice as much fat.

And in animal studies, the evidence is "overwhelming" that a high-fat diet enhances the development of breast tumors, says Clifford Welsch, Ph.D., a tumor biologist with a special interest in breast disease and professor of anatomy at Michigan State University. Dr. Welsch and colleagues are trying to figure out just what it is that links fat with breast disease.

"One idea is that it promotes the secretion of hormones that stimulate the development of both hormone-responsive, normal and cancerous breast tissues," Dr. Welsch says. "It's my opinion that the evidence favors the theory that a high-fat diet increases the susceptibility of the breast tissue to hormone stimulus."

Forty percent of the calories in the average American diet come from fat, mostly in meat and dairy products like butter, cheese and milk. "I think we'd do well to cut that by one-third to one-half," says Dr. Welsch.

And it might be a good idea to replace some of that fat with high-fiber foods, such as whole grains and vegetables. Chronic constipation, something few people eating high-fiber diets experience, has been associated with breast disease.

Researchers at the University of California at San Francisco found that women with severe constipation (two or fewer bowel movements a week) were five times more likely to show signs of possible abnormal cell proliferation in aspirated breast fluids than were women with normal bowel functions.

"It may be that estrogen secreted by the liver is reabsorbed more readily by women with sluggish digestion," says Nicholas Petrakis, M.D., professor of preventive medicine at the University of California,

San Francisco. "This could have a stimulating effect on the breasts."

One other thing the doctors who treat breast disease frequently mention is stress.

"Most of the women I see feel their symptoms are aggravated when they're upset or overworked," Havens says. One of Dr. Love's patients, a politician, only suffers from breast pain when she is campaigning.

"One's attitude, what we call the neuroendocrine aspect of tumorigenesis, can markedly control the development of breast dis-

---

Answers from an Expert

Q: Are there advantages to having small rather than large breasts?

A: No, says Robinson Baker, M.D., director of the Johns Hopkins Breast Clinic in Baltimore. Large-breasted women do not appear to have any greater incidence of breast disease or cancer than small-breasted women, nor need they do anything differently regarding self-examination or mammography.

Q: Does nursing a baby ruin your breasts?

A: It does change the tissue structure of your breasts, giving them less support, so that when you have stopped nursing, your breasts appear somewhat "fallen," Dr. Baker says.

Q: Why do some women find that when they diet, their breasts seem to lose fat first?

A: Breasts are mostly fat, and if you lose weight, you are going to lose fat in your breasts, according to Dr. Baker. While this may seem more noticeable to you, your breasts are not losing fat any faster or sooner than any other part of your body.

Q: Can topless sunbathing harm your breasts?

A: No more than it will the rest of your skin. But if your breasts haven't been exposed to much sunlight, they could burn quickly when exposed, Dr. Baker cautions.

Q: What if you're involved in a contact sport like basketball? Will blows to the breast cause permanent damage?

A: A severe blow could lead to fat necrosis, which can be difficult to distinguish from a tumor because it's very hard. But it will not increase your risk of developing breast disease or cancer, Dr. Baker says.

---

ease," Dr. Welsch says. "It affects the entire central nervous system and can really throw it out of whack."

What's a "good attitude" to have? It's not being so paranoid about getting cancer that you live in fear, but it's also not being negligent about checking your breasts for lumps each month—or taking other measures to reduce the risks, Dr. Welsch says.

CHAPTER 11

Varicose Veins: Relieve the Pressure with Diet and Exercise

Ask your doctor what you can do about varicose veins, and he or she might advise you to choose your parents wisely. "It's an inherited disease," says Robert Nabatoff, M.D., clinical professor of vascular surgery at Mt. Sinai School of Medicine in New York City. "There's really not much you can do to prevent varicose veins. There are 15-year-olds who have them and 80-year-olds who do not have any trace of them. If you're going to get them, you're going to get them."

Not quite so, says another authority. "We don't inherit varicose veins; we inherit a *tendency* to develop varicose veins," says Howard Baron, M.D., attending vascular surgeon at Cabrini Medical Center in New York City and author of *Varicose Veins: A Commonsense Approach to Their Management* (William Morrow). "That's an important distinction."

Indeed, since implicit is the conclusion that varicose veins can be prevented. And whether it's a belief in genetic certainty or some other factor, much of the medical advice on varicose veins deals with treatment rather than prevention. But the truth is that you can do much to prevent the onset of varicose veins, even if you *are* genetically likely to get them. And if you can prevent them for a little while, it follows that you may be able to prevent them for a long while or, perhaps, forever.

Doctors say that exercise, diet and support hosiery are all ways to prevent this affliction, which affects one in four American women and one in ten American men.

Many of us today might think of varicose veins as simply a cosmetic problem, particularly troubling in the summer months when the legs are more exposed in shorts, swim wear and dresses. For some that's the case. For others, however, varicose veins cause fatigue, dull aches in the legs, swelling and sleep-inhibiting cramps. And in a small percentage of cases, complications set in that could be life-threatening, like phlebitis, the development of clots in the deeper veins, and ulceration.

"People who think of varicose veins as only a nuisance are severely underestimating the disease," Dr. Baron says.

A varicose vein is nothing more than a healthy vein gone awry. It didn't start as a varicose vein. It become one. Here's how:

The veins help to transport blood from the legs back to the heart and lungs, where the blood is cleansed of its impurities (carbon dioxide mostly) and refueled with oxygen for another trip through the body. The blood has a more difficult journey from the lower extremities because it's fighting gravity. Fortunately, the leg muscles act like a second heart. As the muscles contract, blood is pumped through the veins. The veins, in turn, are equipped with valves that act like locks on a canal.

The valves allow that blood to flow upward, then snap shut to prevent backward seepage. When the valves are too weak to prevent this gravitational backward flow blood begins to collect in the vein, stretching the vein wall out of shape and producing pain and the often unsightly varicosity. Almost all varicosities occur in the veins near the surface of the leg. Deeper veins are rarely affected because they have support from muscle and fat.

"We inherit a defect in the venous valve or we inherit a vein with a weak or absent wall," Dr. Baron says. "Then there must be an aggravating factor in our lifestyle for the problem to develp. If we avoid aggravating factors, the problem might be delayed or blunted, and it might not develop at all."

Aggravating Factors

The aggravating factors are severe obesity, constipation, standing for prolonged periods, sitting for prolonged periods with legs crossed, and lack of exercise. A common thread runs through all of these factors: They all place added pressure on the surface veins of the legs, increasing the likelihood that varicosities will develop and progress.

Constipation's effect might not be obvious. Because the diets of many Westerners lack sufficient fiber, we tend to suffer from constipation more than people of the so-called Third World who have fiber-rich diets. Even when we're not constipated, our stool tends to be hard and pelletlike and difficult to pass. Both constipation and straining at stool increase intra-abdominal pressure, which is transferred to the veins of the legs. Think of the body as a totem pole with the veins of the lower legs and ankles being the ultimate recipient of pressure from above.

One researcher, in fact, has theorized that constipation and straining at stool are among the primary causes for varicose veins. Denis P. Burkitt, M.D., St. Thomas Hospital Medical School, London, a world-renowned expert on fiber, drew his conclusion after observing tribesmen in Africa who have fiber-rich diets and an exceedingly low incidence of varicose veins.

"It's not only varicose veins. We Americans get other diseases that people with fiber-rich diets don't get, like cancer of the colon and rectum," says Victor Pellicano, M.D., an internist in Lewiston, New York. "In the Western world it's the price we pay for eating so much processed food."

In short, eat more vegetables, fruits and whole grains, and don't strain at stool.

Exercise, too, can head off varicose veins. The flip side, of course, is that lack of exercise exacerbates the problem. "We're a sitting society," says Dr. Baron. "My advice is to walk, run, jog, anything to keep the leg muscles working. Don't sit still. Don't stand still."

Prolonged standing in one place and sitting (particularly with the legs crossed, since that further impedes circulation) allows the blood to pool in the lower extremities. That puts added pressure on a weak valve and can further dilate a vein with a weak wall. Either will hasten the onset of varicose veins. Exercise keeps the body's "second heart," the muscles of the lower legs, contracting and the valves clicking.

The best exercise regimen is to do some activity more often, rather than a lot at one shot. People who are sedentary at work or who are temporarily captive in a plane or a theater can simply press the balls of their feet to the floor to make the calf muscles contract and transport blood. Nothing more elaborate is necessary.

If you have a job that requires that you be on your feet—bartender, beautician, retail clerk—take an elevation break. That is, prop your legs up above your heart several times during the day to allow gravity to speed the blood to the heart.

Support Hosiery and Other Solutions

"Support hosiery is very helpful," Dr. Pellicano says. "Not only does it give comfort to those who already have varicose veins, it could delay the onset of the problem for many years."

Support hosiery exerts graduated pressure on the leg and facilitates blood flow, thus reducing pressure in the veins.

Mass-produced stockings will be fine for most people, but research has shown that for those with great calf-ankle disproportion, hosiery will have to be custom-made to be helpful. For those people, the larger the calf means the hose will have a tourniquet effect and the graduated pressure will be lost.

A few other tips:

• Stop reading on the toilet. The shape of the hardwood or plastic seat puts undue pressure on the abdominal veins, which in turn, put pressure on the leg veins.

•Do not wear any tight garments. particularly calf-length boots, pantyhose too snug at the groin, girdles, corsets and binding belts. All of these tend to constrict venous blood flow.

• Be sure your diet contains orange, tangerines or other citrus fruits. They are a good source of bioflavonoids, which, according to Dr. Pellicano, may delay the onset of varicose veins by strengthening the vein wall, preventing dilation and allowing the valves to work more easily.

The beauty of the doctor's recommendations is that they might stop varicose veins from appearing entirely, or, if they have appeared already, the discomfort may be less acute.

Pregnancy has been linked to varicosities, but it's not causal. Dr. Baron calls pregnancy an "accelerator." What pregnancy does is increase pressure on pelvic veins, much like straining at stool would do, thus obstructing the drainage of blood from the legs.

The pregnancy link has led to the belief that women suffer more from varicose veins than men, and statistics would appear to substantiate that. But Dr. Nabatoff of Mt. Sinai Hospital has an alternative explanation. "Varicose veins are largely a cosmetic thing," he says, "and when women notice them, they're quick to get them treated. Men often ignore the problem. There are plenty of men who have varicose veins. They just don't seek treatment."

Medical Options

If your condition has deteriorated to the point where the varicose veins are large and the pain is becoming more and more of a burden, you might want to consider getting them removed.

"If you have varicose veins and they're not treated, you're 10 times more likely to get phlebitis, clots and ulceration," Dr. Nabatoff says.

"The veins that stick out are susceptible to trauma, irritation and bleeding at the ankle. Almost all ulceration occurs at the ankles." There are two options:

Surgical Removal

This procedure is commonly called "stripping." The varicose veins are tied off and removed. This procedure usually involves an overnight stay in the hospital and several days' rest. But once the vein is gone, so is the varicosity. The condition could possibly recur though, when smaller, previously little-used but diseased veins take over the job of circulating the blood.

The drawbacks to stripping? "Anytime you go under general anesthesia, there's a greater risk and sometimes there's bleeding that can't be controlled without going back in to tie it off," says James DeWeese, M.D., cardiovascular surgeon at the University of Rochester Medical Center.

"The operation is a simple one for any competent vascular surgeon," Dr. Baron says. "And there's a 96 percent cure rate. That means that three years after the operation there is no reappearance of the varicosity in 96 percent of the cases."

Injection Therapy

Done as an office procedure, a chemical solution is injected into the affected vein, causing it to harden and wither away over a period of several months. This procedure works best on smaller varicose veins. "Large varicose veins with high backward pressure don't respond to injection therapy," Dr. Nabatoff says. "If you inject that type, they just recur. The heavy ones you have to tie and strip." With both procedures the patient should be seen again on a yearly basis.

Dr. Baron feels that injection therapy can be dangerous. "What you're doing is forming a chemical phlebitis, and if you're unlucky the clot could extend and make its way into a large vein," he says. Frequently, there are pigment changes at the injection site that are permanent.

It should be clear then that varicose veins are a complex problem. If a close family member has the affliction, you're at risk, but fortunately there's much you can do to prevent the condition. And even if you have varicose veins, preventive measures can help ease your discomfort.

CHAPTER 12

A Menu for Lower Blood Pressure

You begin your day with cantaloupe, freshly squeezed orange juice and bran cereal with skim milk. Lunch is broiled mackerel, parsley potatoes and a salad of watercress, carrot medallions and almonds, tossed with a dressing of fresh garlic in corn oil and apple-cider vinegar. Midafternoon, you calm your rumbling stomach with a cup of low-fat yogurt with banana slices. For dinner, you whip up a luscious casserole of brown rice, onions, broccoli, cashews and melted partly skim mozzarella, lightly spiced with garlic.

If you have high blood pressure, theoretically you've just done everything right. Your one day's menu contains every nutrient known to *lower* blood pressure. Today, medical research has uncovered a way to fight hypertension that's more positive than just avoiding salt and saturated fat. There are actually foods you can eat more of that help you win this often deadly numbers game.

According to Michael Rees, M.D., author of *The Complete Family Guide to Living with High Blood Pressure* (Prentice-Hall), hypertension is the single most important cause of strokes, a major cause of diseases of the heart, brain, kidneys and eyes and, in fact, is the cause of an estimated one-third of all heart disease. Some 60 million Americans have blood pressures that are too high, blood pressures that might just respond to some dietary fine-tuning. They might want to start with this menu:

• **Cantaloupe, winter squash, potatoes, broccoli, orange juice, some fresh fruits and milk.** These are foods containing hefty amounts of potassium. The fact is, how much potassium you have in your diet may be just as important as how little sodium you eat. Studies of vegetarians, who tend to have lower blood pressures than meat eaters, found that their sodium intake was no different from hypertensives but their potassium intake was significantly higher. A group of scientists in Israel looked at the eating habits of 98 vegetarians whose average age was 60 and compared them to a similar group of meat eaters. What they found was a very low prevalence of hypertension—only 2 percent—among the vegetarians although they lived in an adult population where the expected prevalence was 20 to 25 percent. The vegetarians ate as much salt as their neighbors and had the same genetic predisposition to developing hypertension. But they didn't. The researchers concluded that it was their potassium-rich diets of vegetables, fruits and nuts that kept them from developing hypertension (*American Journal of Clinical Nutrition,* May, 1983).

No one really knows potassium protects the body from hypertension even when sodium intake isn't restricted, although there are a number of theories. For one, potassium is an effective diuretic. But in addition to helping the body rid itself of water, potassium also helps slough off sodium too, an effect called natriuresis. Potassium also appears to act on several important physiological systems that regulate blood pressure and control the workings of the vascular system.

In both animal and human studies, potassium seems to have little effect on people whose blood pressures are normal. But it can produce a significant drop in both systolic and diastolic pressures of hypertensives.

And there may be one group of people who benefit most from potassium. According to George R. Meneely, M.D., emeritus professor of medicine at Louisiana State University School of Medicine, there may be "a substantial fraction of the population worldwide, including primitive societies, who develop elevation of the blood pressure if they eat more than four grams of sodium as sodium chloride [normal table salt] a day.

"There is extensive animal evidence," says Dr. Meneely, "that the hypertensogenic [hypertension-causing] effect of excess sodium is counteracted by extra dietary potassium. There is pretty good literature on its effect in humans too."

To avoid potassium loss in cooking, steam rather than boil vegetables. When doctors at a Swedish hospital tested the two cooking methods with potatoes, a rich source of potassium, they discovered that boiled potatoes lose 10 to 50 percent of their potassium while steamed potatoes lost only 3 to 6 percent. They had similar results with carrots, beans and peas (*Lancet,* January 15, 1983).

• **Dairy products, leafy green vegetables like kale and watercress, and nuts.** There's a convincing amount of evidence indicating calcium can lower your blood pressure. Unfortunately, the best sources of calcium—dairy products—also have a fair amount of sodium. A two-ounce serving of Swiss cheese contains 544 milligrams of calcium (the Recommended Dietary Allowance is 800 milligrams), and a hefty 148 milligrams of sodium. But the evidence is too overwhelming in favor of calcium as an antidote to hypertension for anyone to give up milk and cheese entirely. Consider, for example, a study of 82 percent of the adult residents of Rancho Bernardo, an upper-middle-class community in Southern California. What separated the male hypertensives from the normotensives, according to researchers at the University of California, San Diego, was milk. Milk consumption was lower in borderline, untreated and treated hypertensives (*American Journal of Clinical Nutrition,* September, 1983).

In an even larger study, involving 20,749 people across the country, calcium was the only one of 17 nutrients evaluated that differed in the hypertensives. Those people with high blood pressure consumed 18 percent less calcium (*Annals of Internal Medicine,* May, 1983).

That figure alarms researcher David McCarron, M.D., of the division of nephrology and hypertension at the Oregon Health Sciences University in Portland. He conducted that particular study—and several others linking calcium and blood pressure—and he's convinced that a good hypertensive diet has to contain dairy products, sodium and cholesterol notwithstanding.

"If you have to, switch to low-sodium or low-cholesterol cheeses, which are an excellent source of calcium and low in saturated fatty acids," he says. "If you don't have a cholesterol problem and you're near your ideal body weight, you don't necessarily have to worry about the cholesterol."

As for sodium, Dr. McCarron's work indicates that calcium may actually negate the harmful effects of salt on the system. An increased calcium load tends to facilitate the body's excretion of sodium, he notes.

Calcium works on blood pressure in another way—by relaxing the blood vessels. "You'll rarely hear a doctor say that because the most doctors are ever taught in medical school is that calcium makes blood vessels contract," he says. "When blood vessels contract, blood pressure goes up. But calcium actually regulates contraction *and* relaxation of the blood vessels."

But one of the most interesting things to come out of Dr. McCarron's research is not how calcium works alone to lower blood pressure but how it works with potassium, sodium and magnesium to regulate pressure. "It's the proportions of these minerals in the body that seems to be the most important thing," says Dr. McCarron. "The possibility exists that the more you want to eat of one, the more you'd better eat of the others. We, of course, consider calcium the most important. But if you're not taking in enough sodium, potassium and magnesium, the probability is that you're not getting enough calcium either."

And, not coincidentally, the foods that are abundant in one tend to be abundant in the others.

• **Nuts, brown rice, molasses, milk, wheat germ, bananas, potatoes and soy products.** Inadequate dietary magnesium has been shown to increase blood pressure in animals and humans both. Though the exact mechanism isn't known, there is some indication that magnesium exerts its pressure-lowering effect by regulating the entry and exit of calcium in the smooth muscle cells of the vascular system. Together, the two minerals produce the regular contraction and relaxation of blood vessels. In a test involving untreated, newly diagnosed hypertensives, Dr. McCarron found that they consumed less calcium and magnesium than a similar group whose blood pressures were normal. Sodium intake didn't seem to matter (*Annals of Internal Medicine*, May, 1983).

"The interaction of magnesium and calcium gives the calcium the ability to get where it has to in a cell," says Dr. McCarron. "Magnesium facilitates calcium getting to the right place where it can have this relaxing effect."

• **Polunsaturated fats.** In a pilot study of apparently healthy people in Italy, Finland and the United States, researchers discovered that the level of dietary linoleic acid—polyunsaturated fats—was associated with incidence of high blood pressure. There was more hypertensives among the Finnish population than among the Italians and Americans. The Finns consumed more saturated and less polunsaturated fats than the others.

When a group of Finns aged 40 to 50 were placed on a low-fat diet high in polyunsaturated fats and low in saturated fats, even when salt consumption wasn't reduced blood pressures dropped signifcantly. When they returned to their old eating habits, their old blood pressures returned too (*American Journal of Clinical Nutrition,* December, 1983).

James M. Iacono, Ph.D., and other researchers at the U.S. Department of Agriculture Western Human Nutrition Research Center, in San Francisco, believe polunsaturated fats lower blood pressure because, when they're metabolized by the body, they yield a substance that is essential for making prostaglandins. These are fatty acids that seem to control pressure by aiding in the sloughing off of water and salt from the kidneys (*Hypertension,* September/October, 1982).

• **Mackerel and other marine fish high in eicosapentanoic acid, one of the omega-3 fatty acids.** Tests in Germany involving 15 volunteers on a mackerel diet provided some heartening results. After only two weeks, serum tiglycerides and total cholesterol dropped significantly, mirrored by "markedly lower" systolic and diastolic blood pressures.

The Germans were attempting to approximate the diet of Greenland Eskimos and Japanese fishermen, who enjoy a very low incidence of cardiovascular disease. The key appears to be the omega-3 fatty acids found in many fish (*Atheroclerosis,* vol. 49, 1983).

Another study tested the effects of cod-liver oil on the Western diet. Cod-liver oil too contains omega-3 fatty acids. A group of volunteers added three tablespoons of cod-liver oil a day to their normal diets and wound up with lower blood pressures (*Circulation,* March, 1983).

• **Bran, fresh fruits and vegetables, beans and whole grain breads.** The factor here is fiber. There are some early indications from recent tests that plant fiber can significantly lower blood pressure, though precisely why is still a mystery.

Researcher James W. Anderson, M.D., of the Veterans Administration Medical Center in Lexington, Kentucky, placed 12 diabetic men on a 14-day diet containing more than three times the dietary fiber (and fat) of a control diet. Average blood pressures dropped 10 percent. In patients whose blood pressures had been normal, systolic pressures were 8 percent lower and diastolic figures had dropped 10 percent.

The news was even better for the men who had high blood pressure to begin with. Their systolic pressures dropped by 11 percent and diastolic pressure by 10 percent (*Annals of Internal Medicine,* May, 1983).

Dr. Anderson was pleased with his results, but he's not sure why he got them.

"My strongest hunch is that it's related to certain changes in insulin. The patient's insulin needs were low on the high-fiber diet. There's a lot of evidence that insulin contributes to high blood pressure. It's basically a salt-retentive hormone. We also reported a small increase in sodium loss in feces. I didn't think at the time it was meaningful but thinking about it later, having two different mechanisms working together like that—the insulin and the sodium excretion— you can get a synergistic effect."

What makes the results even more significant is that salt use was not restricted during the diet. "In fact," says Dr. Anderson, "there was a 50 percent increase in sodium intake. But potassium also went up, so the sodium:potassium ratio stayed the same."

• **Onions.** The old wives were right. Their tale of onions lowering blood pressure was on target. They do. What the old wives didn't know was why. According to Moses Attrep, Jr., Ph.D., a chemist at East Texas State University, it may be a hormonelike substance he isolated in yellow onions called prostaglandin A_1 which also occurs in the human kidney. When injected into humans and animals, prostaglandin A_1 lowers blood pressure, at least for brief periods.

• **Garlic.** The Japanese and Chinese have used garlic to lower blood pressure for centuries. Its effect is possibly similar to that of onions, since it might also contain prostaglandins. Dr. Attrep is working on an answer to the garlic riddle, too.

CHAPTER 13

The U.S. Male: New Answers for His Special Problems

Although in one way or another many men still play their lives like tough guys in a Humphrey Bogart movie, the truth about men's physical and psychological health is much more complex. There's good evidence that behind the Great Stone Face males are actually weaker than females. Women, it's true, tend to report minor ailments, go to the doctor and worry about their health more than men do. But when men get sick, they're much more likely to get seriously ill and die. Heart attacks, stroke, cancer, atherosclerosis, ulcers: Right down the line, in almost every critical statistic, men fall victim more often than women. The upshot is that the average man can expect to die about eight years sooner than the average woman.

Even nature seems to know the male of the species is more fragile: As many as 170 males are conceived for every 100 females, but because male fetuses are much more likely to die in the womb, by the time of birth the sex ratio is 105 males to every 100 females. Boys' greater vulnerability to infection and genetic diseases continues through childhood, so by the time they reach reproductive age, the numbers have about evened out.

But psychologists argue that this notion of inherent weakness just doesn't explain it all. "An examination of the causes of death of adult men . . . makes the hypothesis of biologic inferiority somewhat suspect," says Kenneth Solomon, M.D., staff psychiatrist at Sheppard and Enoch Pratt Hospital in Baltimore. Most of the leading causes of death among men—heart disease, cancer, stress-related disorders, accidents—are directly or indirectly related to behavior that's traditionally been considered "masculine," he points out.

Society's expectations of men and the traditional male way of dealing with the pressure seem designed to cook up a bubbling stew of inner stress. Men are taught to fight for success, status and achievement—at the same time they're barred from showing any signs of uncertainty or weakness. They're encouraged to be daring, violent, aggressive and unafraid of risk. They're supposed to be tough and confident, know all the answers—and do it all alone.

"Anything that is remotely or vaguely feminine, whether it be in role, behavior, thought or feeling," is strictly taboo, Dr. Solomon says. As a result, men are limited in the way they can deal with stressful situations—so most of them just bottle it up. "Women tend to acknowledge that they're under stress, what's producing the stress, and what feelings this situation produces," says Dr. Solomon "Men tend to deny

---

Psychological Self-Care

Men could do their physical health a favor by altering some traditionally male psychological patterns, says psychologist Herb Goldberg, Ph.D. Some of his suggestions:

1. Learn to listen to what your body is saying, and learn to respond to what it tells you. Your body's messages of pain or pleasure, hunger or fatigue are your guideposts to survival. To ignore, deny or disguise them is to risk irreversible damage to your health.

2. Learn to cherish the joys of rest. When you're tired, take a nap. When you're not feeling well or you're overworked, go to bed. Learn to delight in sleeping—it's not "unmale" or a waste of time.

3. Learn to separate masculinity from a meat-centered diet. You can be just as much of a man with a salad as with a steak—and you may even feel better when you're through.

4. Learn to be a little more vain, at least when it comes to your body. Spend some time each day grooming and observing yourself in the mirror. Praise yourself when you like what you see; respond with alarm and positive action when you don't.

5. Find an older man who is in great shape and, even if your first impulse is to dismiss him as a fanatic, find out how he does it. Don't be proud. Ask questions. He may know something you don't know—and if your health benefits, you win.

and bury the whole thing. They adopt a very unemotional, rational, problem-solving sort of attitude. They tend not to even know they're under stress."

Result? Stress-related illnesses like peptic ulcers, high blood pressure and heart disease are epidemic among men.

Men also drink and smoke more, and drive less prudently than women do—partly as a way of handling stress, partly because it's considered "masculine."

Men, clearly, are under pressure, and the pressure tightens its squeeze on their physical health because so many of them have simply lost touch with their bodies, says Francis Baumli, Ph.D., a medical consultant who writes extensively on men's issues. "Men tend to ignore minor health problems until they become major ones," he says. "Far too often, the first time they call attention to the problem is in the emergency room rather than the consulting room of the family doctor."

In many ways, the blame for this can be laid at the foot of traditional male role conditioning, says Herb Goldberg, Ph.D., a psychologist and author of *The New Male* (Signet). "Boys are taught very early in life that it's unmanly to be ill, unmanly to complain, and unmanly to ask for help," he says. Admitting being sick also means being passive and dependent—and sick in bed is no place for a real man.

Dr. Goldberg also points to the psychological defense of "intellectualization" as a reason for men's dangerous inability to hear what their bodies are saying. "By intellectualization I mean the kind of orientation to one's body and health that in effect says 'I will accept it as true only if you can prove it to me objectively with scientific data or if it is spoken by an authority in the field.'" That's not an objection to the scientific approach itself, he says, but to a state of affairs where we are "so out of touch with our bodies that we constantly must consult an authority figure to know what to do with them." The sad result, he says, is that "a man may 'feel great' one day and suffer a heart attack the next. I always wonder when I hear of such instances, where were the body's messages of distress all during the time it was weakening to the point of this total collapse?"

Becoming a Better Man

But if the American male is out of touch with his own body, beset by stress, full of bottled-up tension and bound for an early grave, what's he supposed to do about it? "Men are simply going to have to learn to take it easy—and that's not going to be easy," Dr. Solomon says. "They're going to have to learn that there's more to life than working, that 'success' is killing them." In some ways, he adds, the women's movement is going to force men to change for the better by becoming more relaxed and sensitive husbands, and more equal partners in the role of parents. "But I think women are still protecting the 'fragile male ego' too much. I think they need to more openly encourage men to change."

Very often, Dr. Baumli says, since men tend to ignore or deny their illnesses, it becomes their wives' responsibility to point out the seriousness of their symptoms and get them to go to the doctor—or to stop doing whatever it is that's causing the problem. "Women often become a sort of 'health motivator' for their men." But this pattern, too, needs to change: Men need to take charge of their own bodies and their own health. And in many ways, the tremendous renaissance of interest in health and fitness has demonstrated that men *are* beginning to do that. The death rate from heart disease—traditionally a "man's problem" —has actually declined in recent years.

The Trouble with the Prostate

One thing that *hasn't* seemed to decline is that male annoyance, the prostate problem. If there's any part of the male body that seems designed for no other purpose than to cause trouble, it's the prostate. An estimated 12 million American men, most of them over 40, have some kind of trouble with this gland; by the time a man reaches 85, he has a 95 percent chance of having to share his old age with an enlarged prostate.

Normally a chestnut-sized gland whose primary known function is to supply the liquid part of a man's ejaculate, the prostate can swell up to the size of an orange. Since it completely surrounds the urethra, or urinary exit pipe, it's not hard to understand what happens when it swells. (Two men were sharing a hospital room, the story goes. "Wwwwhat's your tr-tr-trouble?" one asked. "Prostate," the other replied. "I used to pee the way you talk.")

Benign prostate hypertrophy (BPH), or noncancerous enlargement of the prostate, is a common problem. It's not clear what causes it, but it's so widespread among older men it's thought that age-related hormonal changes are a major factor. Another potential—and preventable—culprit: fatty diets. Autopsies of enlarged human prostates have shown an extraordinarily high cholesterol content compared with normal prostates, and experiments with dogs have shown that reducing dietary cholesterol may reduce the size of a swollen prostate.

BPH, while little more than painful and annoying, may be paving the way for something far worse: cancer. In a study involving almost 1,200 case histories, researchers found that the death rate from prostate cancer was three to seven times higher among men with BPH than health controls (*Lancet,* July 20, 1974).

Another major kind of prostate problem is prostatitis. Symptoms range from acute pain and fever to cloudy discharges and painful urination. It's caused by bacterial infections or (much more commonly) an unknown agent, and the traditional medical approach is to drop a depth charge of broad-spectrum antibiotics in hopes that something will hit. But it's also been known for 50 years that zinc is essential to the health of the prostate, and the prostatic fluid itself is extraordinarily high in the mineral. Irving Bush, M.D., professor of urology at the Chicago Medical School, has found that men with chronic prostatis generally have low zinc levels in both prostate fluid and semen, and that patients with prostate cancer also have low zinc stores.

Oral zinc sulfate, he and his colleagues have found, may help resolve prostatitis. In one study, 200 patients with infectious prostatis were given between 11 and 34 milligrams of zinc daily for up to 16 weeks. All registered higher semen levels of zinc—and 70 percent reported relief from their symptoms. Zinc seemed to help patients with BPH, too. A total of 250 BPH patients received 34 milligrams of oral zinc a day for two months and then started a long-term program of 11 to 23 milligrams daily. Eighty percent reported some easing of their symptoms, 25 percent had an increased urine flow, and 20 percent showed an actual decrease in prostate size. It's not clear how zinc does its little dance on the prostate, since other studies at Washington University School of Medicine in St. Louis, have shown that oral zinc raises serum (blood) zinc levels but doesn't raise the level in the prostate itself.

Certainly the most serious of all prostate problems is cancer—the second most common type of cancer among men and a scourge that kills about 20,000 Americans annually. Strangely, quite a few of these cancers are very slow growing, and doctors who find them in older men often just leave them alone—the cure is worse than the disease. But for men hit by the aggressive, fast-spreading kind of malignancy, prompt diagnosis and treatment is critical. If caught early, the 10-year cure rate for these cancers is almost 100 percent. Unfortunately, only about 10 percent of prostate cancers are discovered before they've spread beyond the organ itself. That's why the best kind of prevention for prostate cancer, especially for men over 50, is an annual rectal exam.

Testicular Cancer: Rare but Deadly

Another potential health problem unique to the male is cancer of the testes. It's actually fairly rare, accounting for only about 1 percent of all cancers in men, but among males under 35, it's one of the most common malignancies. A 1976 National Cancer Institute report also showed that its incidence is increasing, and that it's striking men earlier in life. Prompt diagnosis and treatment can cure almost all testicular cancers, but few men actually received that treatment.

A recent study at Massachusetts General Hospital looked at the medical care received by 133 men with testicular cancer and found that more than 60 percent weren't treated promptly, either because they delayed seeking therapy or because their condition was misdiagnosed by their doctor. (Most common misdiagnoses: epididymitis, or inflammation or the testes, or physical injury to the testes.) Of those who weren't treated promptly, 29 percent died as a result of their disease.

George Prout, M.D., chief of urology at Massachusetts General, hospital, says virtually all testicular cancers can be cured if they're treated within a month of symptoms. To detect these cancers while they're still treatable, Dr. Prout recommends that all men perform a simple testicular self-exam once a month. Though not all malignancies can be felt, many will feel like a hard lump or nodule in the testes, or the testes may become enlarged. Any enlargement that lasts longer than three weeks and doesn't respond to antibiotics should be considered cancerous and removed, Dr. Prout says. That's the price of the cure: surgical removal of the testes, followed by chemotherapy. But which would you rather lose—your testicles or your life?

Vasectomy: A Health Risk?

Among men who've decided to become sterile, vasectomy has become an increasingly common choice. About half a million American men are sterilized by vasectomy annually. But in recent years there have been some worrisome reports about long-term health risks associated with vasectomy, especially an increased risk of atherosclerosis. Studies published in the late 1970's showed that vasectomized monkeys fed a high-fat, high-cholesterol diet were more likely to develop atherosclerosis than nonvasectomized monkeys eating the same kind of food. But more recent studies have concluded—though it's still unclear—why the operation doesn't pose the same risks to humans. One group of researchers followed 4,733 vasectomized men for a combined total of over 33,000 man-years and found that the risk of nonfatal heart attack was almost identical to that of a much larger group of nonvasectomized men. "This long-term follow-up study provides substantial reassurance that the risk of acute myocardial infarction [heart attack] is not increased in men [less than or equal to] 15 years after vasectomy," they concluded (*Journal of Urology,* November, 1983).

"The bottom line is that vasectomy doesn't appear to cause any serious long-term side effects at all, whether it be heart disease, autoimmune diseases, cancer or neurological disorders," says Sherman Silber, M.D., a fertility specialist at St. Luke's West Hospital in St. Louis and author of *How to Get Pregnant* (Warner Books). "It's a pretty safe procedure."

That's not to say that vasectomy doesn't cause some *minor* health problems, he says. It's not uncommon for vasectomized men to complain of some pain in the testicles, he says, and about 10 percent of the time the pain persists. It's usually caused by congestive epididymitis, or a swelling of the blocked-up sperm ducts (which lie on the surface of the testes), or by sperm granulomas, hardened masses of tissues that grow up around semen that leaks from the vasectomy site. "Actually, when you look at those tubules under a microscope and see all the damage vasectomy causes, it's amazing it doesn't hurt more," Dr. Silber says. But most men don't feel anything, and 99 percent express overall satisfaction with the operation, he adds.

Testicular Self-Exam

1. The best time for this simple three-minute self-exam is right after a warm bath or shower, when the skin of the scrotum is most relaxed and the testicles are easiest to feel.

2. Examine the testicles separately, using the fingers of both hands. Put your index and middle fingers underneath the testicle and your thumb on top. Then gently roll the testicle between thumb and fingers. If it hurts, you're applying too much pressure.

3. A normal testicle is oval, somewhat firm to the touch, and should be smooth and free of lumps. On the back side of each testicle you'll feel the epididymis (sperm storage duct), which is a little spongier to the touch.

4. What you're looking for—and hoping not to find—is a small, hard, usually painless lump or swelling on the front or side of the testicle. If you do, have it checked by a doctor right away.

5. It's a good idea to do this exam at least once a month.

If he were performing a vasectomy on any of his friends, Dr. Silber explains he'd do an "open-ended" operation, a less common procedure that reduces the risk of minor pain and swelling. By not completely sealing off one of the severed ends of the vas deferens, or sperm duct, pressure in the duct itself doesn't "blow out" the cordlike epididymis's delicate plumbing along the testes and cause the dull ache some men complain of. But to prevent the risk of surprise pregnancy, the end of the vas leading to the penis must be very securely sealed.

Zinc for Fertility

For other men, the price of *in*fertility is even higher: the inability to have a child of one's own. In fact, about a sixth of all married couples in the United States—3½ million of them—are infertile (that is, they've tried to produce a pregnancy for at least a year without success). Traditionally, and unfairly, infertility was thought of as a woman's problem. But fertility specialists now believe that about 40 percent of the time it's the man's reproductive system that's to blame.

The fundamental problem is that there's been an alarming and steady decline in sperm counts among American males since the 1920's. Over the past 20 years, studies of large numbers of sperm donors have recorded a drop in the average sperm count of almost 50 percent. Often, Dr. Silber told us, there are congenital problems with sperm production in the testicle itself; sometimes a varicose vein in the testes interferes with sperm production by raising the organ's temperature (this can be fixed surgically); sometimes the epididymis is blocked by infection.

But the underlying cause of these problems remains unclear. Dr. Silber speculates that stress could be the cause, somehow interfering with hormones that control sperm production. Others blame toxic chemicals, to which the male reproductive system is especially sensitive. One study at Florida State University in 1979 turned up alarmingly low sperm counts in semen samples from 132 student volunteers—23 had levels so low they were effectively sterile—as well as high levels of four toxic chemicals, including DDT and PCB's.

But whatever is bringing sperm counts down, there is no magic medicine that will bring them up again. "For years we have looked for some hormonal treatment, similar to inducing ovulation in women, that might improve sperm count, but the results have frequently been disappointing," Dr. Silber says.

If you are having trouble producing a longed-for conception, there are a few safe, natural things you can try, though. One is zinc, a mineral known to be especially important to a man's reproductive system. It's been shown to increase the motility (movement) of sperm, and is present in high amounts in healthy semen and prostatic fluid. Nuts, sunflower seeds, eggs, whole grains, milk, peas and carrots are all good sources of zinc.

Although not a common problem, male infertility caused by sperm agglutination ("clumping up") may be helped dramatically by vitamin C, a University of Texas study had shown. Fifteen men who were unable to impregnate their wives were found to have extremely high rates of sperm agglutination (an average of 37 percent, where 20 percent is considered the threshold of infertility) as well as low semen levels of vitamin C. Researchers prescribed 500 milligram of vitamin C twice a day (a gram daily, total), and in only four days their average agglutination rate had dropped to 20 percent. In a week, it dropped to 14 percent and in three weeks to 11 percent (*Journal of the American Medical Association,* May 27, 1983).

Also: Don't smoke anything—both tobacco and marijuana can reduce sperm counts. Avoid unnecessary x-rays, which can do the same. And drink alcohol only in moderation, since alcohol can reduce the male sex hormone testosterone. Some commonly prescribed medications may also affect male fertility. The ulcer drug Tagamet, for instance, has been shown to reduce sperm counts significantly (they return to normal once the drug is discontinued), and the antidepressant lithium carbonate can reduce sperm viability.

CHAPTER 14

Answers to Your Most Embarrassing Health Problems

When you're really sick, you can at least expect to get some sympathy. But if you suffer from gas, bad breath, smelly feet or any number of other physical faux pas, you're more likely to get nasty looks than kind words.

While these social ailments won't outright kill you, they might embarrass you enough to wish you were dead, at least at the moment.

But you don't have to put up with your body's annoying habits. Even the worst problems can have simple solutions.

The Incredible Exploding Stomach

Taking baking soda to induce a burp and relieve your stuffed stomach could make things worse, much worse. In five cases, baking soda has literally burst a stomach apart. When the alkaline mixture hits stomach acid, the result is truly explosive.

One recent case involved a 31-year-old man who downed two margaritas, an order of nachos and a large combination platter at a Mexican restaurant. He then went home and drank a half teaspoon of baking soda in a half glass of water. Within minutes his stomach ruptured. Emergency surgery saved his life.

Bathroom Roulette

How would you like to be the guy who has just touched down in a foreign country and is riding into town when he just *knows* he's "gotta go"?

First he has to convince the hardnosed bus driver that his vehicle will never be the same unless he stops immediately. Then, he must race to the nearest cottage and beg to use the facilities. For years, doctors told this man his problem was "irritable bowel syndrome" brought on by nerves. It's true that stress can be a major cause of diarrhea. But this man discovered milk was his problem. More specifically, lactose intolerance—the inability to digest milk sugar.

"Many people don't relate their chronic diarrhea to milk because the symptoms are delayed. They don't appear until three to six hours after eating," says Chesley Hines, M.D., of the Ochsner Clinic in New Orleans.

Check, too, for other common culprits—coffee, alcohol, chocolate, too much sugar (especially in children) and some artificial sweeteners.

Try eating more fiber. Both bran and pectin help soak up runny stools and prevent too-fast passage.

And watch for antibiotic-caused diarrhea. These drugs knock out good bacteria in the bowel and allow toxin-producing bad guys to take over. The result can be bowel problems that last for months.

Acidophilus, a friendly bacteria normally found in the bowel, can relieve these symptoms, says Richard Huemer, M.D., of Westlake Village, California. "I've found that two acidophilus capsules just before meals helps restore the normal bacterial environment in the intestine."

Taming Bean Power

Beans are an almost universal gas producer. They contain starches that ferment in the bowel. Degas your beans this way: Soak them for three hours, boil for about 30 minutes (add fresh water if needed) and discard water.

Here's a flatulence rating for beans, starting with the most powerful.

soybeans	Great Northern beans
pink beans	baby limas
black beans	garbanzos
pinto beans	large limas
California small	black-eyed peas
white beans	

Laugh at Your Own Risk

Do you dribble urine when you giggle? Gush when you guffaw? If so, you may be a victim of common female malady—stress incontinence.

Mild symptoms respond well to exercises that strengthen the muscles that form a figure 8 around the vagina and anus and close the urethra opening, says Zafar Khan, M.D., director of the Urodynamics Lab at Beth Israel Medical Center in New York City. Try tensing these muscles for a few seconds as you would to stop urine flow. Then relax. Build up to 50 to 100 contractions a day.

Using biofeedback to learn to keep these muscles contracted when pressure is felt has worked well in an experimental program at Johns Hopkins Medical Center, in Baltimore. "Biofeedback combined with exercises at home reduced our patient's frequency of incontinence by 80 percent," says program director William Whitehead, Ph.D.

Air-Robics We Can Do Without

Real men do it, sitting in front of the TV set, beer in hand. And they don't cover their mouths, either.

It's normal to belch once or twice after a big meal, says Dr. Michael Levitt, M.D. Your stomach is releasing air you've swallowed along with your food. A belch relieves fullness and makes you feel better.

Eating quickly or while you're anxious, talking with your mouth full, and slurping soup can all increase belching. So can carbonated drinks, gum chewing, a stuffy nose or poor-fitting dentures.

But most big belchers create their own problem, Dr. Levitt says. "They have gotten into the nervous habit of swallowing air, and once they realize what they're doing, they can't easily stop it."

Kiss Your Cold Sores Goodbye

It's hard enough to face the real world some days, much less do it with a giant cold sore nibbling at your lip. What can you do? Try taking lysine, says Mark McCune, M.D., an Overland Park, Kansas, dermatologist who treats both cold sores and genital herpes with this essential amino acid.

In several studies, lysine cut the incidence of herpes breakouts, sometimes completely eliminating them. "It relieves burning, reduces the spread of blistering, and seems to speed healing in some people," Dr. McCune says.

But make sure you're getting enough to keep your herpes at bay. "Take at least 1,000 milligrams a day," warns Dr. McCune.

And put zinc oxide ointment on your cold sores at night. "Zinc is a known antiviral agent, and it seems to speed healing," Dr. McCune says. Dr. Huemer adds another suggestion: adequate vitamin C and A, and zinc.

Scratch Itching Off Your List

One of the worst tortures is itching in a place that's too private to scratch openly. Rubbing up against doorknobs or desk corners might provide temporary relief, but it could also give you a reputation.

Skin that itches without a rash is often dry, says Morris Waisman, M.D., a Tampa, Florida, dermatologist. The initial itching may be caused by too scrupulous skin care, especially hot soapy soaks, that people take even more frequently as their itching increases.

Take fewer baths, especially during dry winter months, Dr. Waisman says. Use tepid water and go easy on the soap. Smooth on a skin oil or lotion to seal in moisture when you step from the tub.

An itchy bottom can also be the result of trying to be too clean, particularly in women, Dr. Waisman says. Avoid using soap, which can be quite irritating.

Vaginal yeast infections cause severe itching and require a doctor's attention.

Jock itch can also be a yeast infection, or ringworm. Athlete's foot can sometimes spread to the genitals.

Itching around the anus can be a fungus infection, hemorrhoids, allergic contact or a reaction to spicy foods, Dr. Waisman says. You'll need medication for an infection. For hemorrhoids, try witch hazel or a topical cream that stops itching.

In all three cases, wear roomy cotton briefs that don't trap sweat or heat. Make sure your detergent or fabric softener, or your toilet paper, isn't causing your itch.

When the Breathalizer Refuses *You*

Does your wife cringe when you kiss her? How about your dog?

Bad breath may be the most feared social disease. It's nearly impossible to tell if you have it—you can't smell your own breath—and who wants to tell someone else he does?

Bad breath is often caused by "blowing air over something that doesn't smell good," says Michale Lerner, D.D.S., a Lexington, Kentucky, dentist with a special interest in nutrition. That "something" may be a gum infection packed with odor-producing bacteria. Get your gum disease treated and brush and floss carefully to prevent further problems. And take vitamins C, A and bioflavonoids to strengthen gum tissue, Dr. Lerner says.

Guess what else is loaded with bacteria? Your tongue. In fact, deadly morning breath is the work of sulfur-producing bacteria. Give them the brush-off with your toothbrush. One dental researcher found that brushing your tongue along with the teeth reduced odor-causing breath gases by 85 percent.

Smelly Feet

Do people run away screaming when they see you untying your shoelaces? Maybe it's their way of hinting that you have lethally offensive feet. Most people need to have someone else point this out to them, says Harvey Lemont, D.P.M., of the Philadelphia College of Podiatric Medicine.

Often, feet smell because they sweat too much. Sweat promotes rapid growth of normal foot bacteria, and the bacteria break down dead skin cells, producing chemicals with that "dead sneaker" scent.

Emotional upsets, drugs, diabetes, and obesity can all cause sweaty feet, but often no underlying reason can be found and people can only treat their symptoms, Dr. Lemont says.

Keep your feet dry. Stick to cotton or wool socks, and change them often. Wear only leather shoes, and give them a chance to dry out every other day by alternating pairs. Soak your feet in an aluminum salts bath, which will make them sweat less. Scrub off dead skin and use a medicated powder on your feet, socks and shoes.

A new over-the-counter foot deodorant, Lavilin, practically eliminated foot odor in 34 out of 35 patients treated for this problem by podiatrist Marc Brenner, president of the American Society of Podiatric Dermatology. "It appears to eliminate odor by destroying bacteria on the skin surface and seems to be nonirritating and safe to use," he says.

Rodale Press, Inc., publishes PREVENTION®, the better health magazine.
For information on how to order your subscription,
write to PREVENTION®, Emmaus, PA 18049.